Successful Online Learning

Managing the Online Learning Environment Efficiently and Effectively

EDITED BY

Theresa A. Middleton Brosche, MSN, BSN, RN, CCRN
Adjunct Instructor
State University of New York–Delhi
Delhi, New York

Staff RN
Mary Washington Hospital
Fredericksburg, Virginia

Adjunct Clinical Faculty
Germanna Community College
Locust Grove, Virginia

Michelle Feavel, MSN, RN
Houston, Texas

JONES AND BARTLETT PUBLISHERS
Sudbury, Massachusetts
BOSTON TORONTO LONDON SINGAPORE

World Headquarters
Jones and Bartlett Publishers
40 Tall Pine Drive
Sudbury, MA 01776
978-443-5000
info@jbpub.com
www.jbpub.com

Jones and Bartlett Publishers Canada
6339 Ormindale Way
Mississauga, Ontario L5V 1J2
Canada

Jones and Bartlett Publishers International
Barb House, Barb Mews
London W6 7PA
United Kingdom

Jones and Bartlett's books and products are available through most bookstores and online booksellers. To contact Jones and Bartlett Publishers directly, call 800-832-0034, fax 978-443-8000, or visit our website, www.jbpub.com.

Substantial discounts on bulk quantities of Jones and Bartlett's publications are available to corporations, professional associations, and other qualified organizations. For details and specific discount information, contact the special sales department at Jones and Bartlett via the above contact information or send an email to specialsales@jbpub.com.

Production Credits
Publisher: Kevin Sullivan
Acquisitions Editor: Emily Ekle
Acquisitions Editor: Amy Sibley
Associate Editor: Patricia Donnelly
Editorial Assistant: Rachel Shuster
Senior Production Editor: Carolyn F. Rogers
Marketing Manager: Rebecca Wasley
V.P., Manufacturing and Inventory Control: Therese Connell
Composition: Shepherd, Inc.
Cover Design: Kristin E. Parker
Cover Images: background © Octus/ShutterStock, Inc.; laptop with screens © nmedia/ShutterStock, Inc.
Printing and Binding: Malloy, Inc.
Cover Printing: Malloy, Inc.

Library of Congress Cataloging-in-Publication Data
Brosche, Theresa Ann Middleton.
Successful online learning : managing the online learning environment efficiently and effectively / Theresa Ann Middleton Brosche and Michelle Feavel.
p. cm.
ISBN 978-0-7637-7619-0 (pbk.)
1. Distance education—United States. 2. Educational technology—United States. 3. Web-based instruction. I. Feavel, Michelle. II. Title.
LB2328.15.U6B76 2010
371.33'44678—dc22
2009032446

6048

Printed in the United States of America
13 12 11 10 09 10 9 8 7 6 5 4 3 2 1

For "Mama Chick" Susie Sonnier,

For the times you made us see beyond our own struggles,
For the times you helped us get through just one more class,
For the times you talked us through wanting to give up or give in.
But most of all, for bringing us together as friends . . .

Terry, Michelle, Julie, Debbie, Desi, Elizabeth, Patti, Stacia,
Sally, Chad, Kathleen, Laura, and Sherry

"Life is what we make it. Always has been, always will be."

—Grandma Moses

Contents

Preface

This concise, practical, and easy-to-use handbook will serve as a reference and a resource for students who are new to the online learning environment, students who are considering the online learning environment, and students who already enrolled in the online learning environment. What makes this handbook unique are the real-life scenarios, strategies and tips for success, and checklists at the end of each chapter, written with the hopes of helping the student to function efficiently and effectively in the online learning environment. What also makes this handbook unique is that each contributing author has been or is currently engaging in the online learning environment as a student or a faculty member. The information presented in each chapter, therefore, is based on firsthand experiences along with a unique awareness of what the online learner needs to assist in minimizing obstacles in this learning environment and includes the following:

- Communicating
- Identifying learning styles
- Dealing with expected and unexpected challenges
- Working in groups
- Setting up an ergonomically sound workspace
- Writing and formatting papers
- Encouraging collegiality
- Managing the first day of the course
- Overcoming technological barriers and concerns
- Taking a look at online learning from the faculty perspective

We hope you enjoy the handbook, and we hope that it helps to make your online learning experience a memorable one.

Theresa Ann Middleton Brosche and Michelle Feavel

Foreword

This book provides an excellent window into the ever-growing world of online learning. Students need a better understanding of online learning communities and their roles and responsibilities in these communities. This useful handbook provides students with effective solutions and strategies for effective online learning. Online education books tend to focus on what the faculty needs to do or how to develop online courses. These are important areas, but students need resources as they make decisions to participate in online learning and then a guide to finding their way around this new learning environment. This book does this for online students. The reader is drawn into the content with short real-life examples and experiences. The book includes tips that can be easily applied and provides rationales for how the tips can support effective learning. The authors include challenges that are not so uncommon when a student takes an online course, such as weather that shuts down the electricity or a death in the family. From practical technical tips to guides on how to work with fellow students in the online learning environment, the online student is the focus. A recent report from the U.S. Department of Education indicates that "on average students in online learning conditions performed better than those receiving face-to-face instruction" (2009, p. ix). To accomplish this, students need to learn much more about online learning and strategies to be effective online learners. This handbook will help students be successful.

Anita Finkelman, MSN, RN
Dean of Online Education
Galen College of Nursing

Reference

U.S. Department of Education, Office of Planning, Evaluation, and Policy Development. (2009). *Evaluation of evidence-based practices in online education: A meta-analysis and review of online learning studies*. Washington, DC: Author.

Contributors

Editor
Theresa A. Middleton Brosche, MSN, RN, CCRN
Adjunct Faculty, Germanna Community College, Locust Grove, Virginia
Adjunct Faculty, State University of New York (SUNY), online RN-BSN
Walden University Graduate

Contributing Editor
Michelle Feavel, MSN, RN
Retired
Walden University Graduate

Contributing Authors
Anita C. All, RN, PhD
Professor and Director, Auburn University/Auburn Montgomery joint MSN program, Auburn, Alabama
Wachovia Endowed Professor

Theresa A. Middleton Brosche, MSN, BSN, RN, CCRN
Adjunct Faculty, Germanna Community College, Locust Grove, Virginia
Adjunct Faculty, State University of New York (SUNY), online RN-BSN
Walden University Graduate

Desiree D. Carter, MSN, RN
Section Instructor, Florida Hospital College of Health Sciences online program
Adjunct Faculty, State University of New York (SUNY), online RN-BSN
Walden University Graduate
Nominating Committee Chairperson for the Walden University Nursing Alumni Association, 2009–2010

Patricia A. Clayburn, MSN, RN
Assistant Professor, MedCentral College of Nursing, Mansfield, Ohio
Walden University Graduate

Michelle Feavel, MSN, RN
Retired
Walden University Graduate

Julie Fomenko, MSN, RN
Clinical Assistant Professor, Texas A & M University–Corpus Christi
Walden University Graduate

Michael R. George
Instructional Technologist, Fredericksburg City Public Schools
MEd Curriculum and Instruction—George Mason University

Patricia Lisk, MS, DACCE
Professor of Nursing
Germanna Community College, Locust Grove, Virginia

Elizabeth L. Pratt, MSN, RNC
Assistant Professor of Nursing, Southern Arkansas University, Magnolia, Arkansas
Adjunct Faculty, State University of New York (SUNY), online RN-BSN
Walden University Graduate
Member of the Walden University Alumni Association

Katherine Quartuccio, MSN/ED, RN
Adjunct Faculty, Germanna Community College, Locust Grove, Virginia
University of Phoenix Graduate

Sally Rudy, MSN, RN
Simulation Nurse Educator, Penn State Hershey Medical Center, Hershey, Pennsylvania
Walden University Graduate

Deborah Schlief, MSN, RNC, IBCLC
Clinical Educator, NCH Healthcare System, Naples, Florida
Clinical Associate, Edison State College, Naples, Florida
Walden University Graduate
Member of the Walden University Alumni Association

Susan Sonnier, MS, RN
Adjunct Faculty, State University of New York (SUNY), online RN-BSN
Patient Education Coordinator, Clear Lake Regional Medical Center, Webster, Texas
Walden University Graduate
Walden University Nursing Alumni Association—Founding Member and Vice President, 2007–2008; Membership Chairman, 2008–2009

Stacia Thompson, MSN, RN
Associate Professor, Iowa Western Community College, Council Bluffs, Iowa
Walden University Graduate

Chad Troxell, MSN, RN
Adjunct Instructor, Florida Hospital College of Health Sciences online program
House Supervisor, Santa Rosa Medical Center, Milton, Florida
Walden University Graduate
Vice-President of the Walden University Nursing Alumni Association

Chapter 1

Even a "Technopeasant" Can Succeed in Online Learning Programs!

Desiree Carter

A comedian once performed a skit during which he referred to himself as a "technopeasant." *Technopeasant* is a neologism used to describe individuals who lack knowledge about computers, are unwilling to use computers, and/or are resistant to keeping up with rapidly advancing technology. There is no denying that computers and related technology are central to current, everyday life, providing a wide variety of new opportunities for a vast cross-section of our population. One such opportunity is online learning, which opens doors for those who may not have otherwise had the chance to further their education.

However technologically challenged an individual may be, it is possible to approach and engage in the online learning experience and succeed. A wealth of online educational programs exist, ranging from those that are designed for students who are novices at computer usage to those who consider themselves experienced and expertly capable. This chapter will explore the technology used in the online learning environment, review similarities between online and traditional education, and examine myths concerning an online course of study. Tips on how to get started and how to minimize the bumps in the road of an online program are also provided.

Confessions of a True Technopeasant!

I graduated with both an associate's degree and a bachelor's degree in nursing from traditional educational programs. When I started to consider an online program to obtain my master's degree, I did not even know how to attach a document to an email. I discussed this with the school recruiter and was assured that there would be tutorials available to help me with all of the skills necessary for success in the program. As a result of my online learning program, I now have a solid grasp of computer skills, and I am not afraid to try new things. I am a true picture of a recovering technopeasant!

The Online Learning Environment

Online education is based on the constructivism learning theory (Holly, Legg, Mueller, & Adelman, 2008; Wambach et al., 1999). The guiding principles of this theory place an emphasis on the learner being an active participant in the learning process, and the educator, or the instructor, primarily serving as a facilitator. The students accept the responsibility for learning through a collaborative relationship with the educator and with other students through various types of assignments. By accepting the responsibility for learning and possessing a degree of confidence and self-direction in the learning process, Ryan and colleagues assert that the students will be able to concentrate on learning and not be intimidated by computers due to a lack of exposure or skills (Ryan, Carlton, & Ali, 2004).

Exploration of Technology and Tips on How to Get Started

A student who chooses to engage in the online learning experience must honestly assess his or her computer knowledge and skills prior to enrolling in an online program. It is also helpful to have a basic understanding of frequently used computer programs such as Microsoft Word, Adobe Acrobat Reader, and Microsoft PowerPoint:

- Microsoft Word is a word processing program commonly utilized for writing papers and other documents.
- Adobe Acrobat Reader is a software program for viewing and printing PDF documents (Wambach et al., 1999). Many academic journals utilize Adobe Acrobat Reader because it preserves the integrity of the contents of the documents by not allowing anyone other than the author to alter the original document.
- Microsoft PowerPoint is a presentation program that enables the user to develop a written presentation with slides that can include text, pictures, charts, graphs, and video. Faculty often use Microsoft PowerPoint to develop written presentations of their lectures (Holly et al., 2008; Ryan et al., 2004).

Those who possess minimal or limited skills should take the time to review the computer literacy requirements for participation in the program. Basic computer skills, such as accessing the Internet, signing into the classroom, and using tabs or radio buttons that allow one to maneuver in the online classroom are essential components of virtually all online learning environments. Additional skills include downloading and uploading documents to and from the computer.

Downloading documents entails retrieving a document from another source and saving it on to your computer. Uploading documents involves sending a document as an attachment from your computer to another location. In the online learning environment, this other location could be a drop box or a discussion board that enables instructors and/or students to view the document. One easy way you can learn to download and upload documents is by sending your friends emails that contain some type of attachment, and then have these friends send emails back to you with attachments so you can practice saving them to a personal file.

All of these skill sets enable you to communicate with the instructor and classmates and vice versa, so their importance becomes obvious. Allow yourself time to become comfortable with these skills before access to and navigation of the program becomes imperative.

If you find that mastering these basic skill sets is an issue, a conversation with the program advisor before you begin your coursework is appropriate to evaluate the potential need for tutorials or other assistance. Remember, simply because you do not possess certain computer skills does not mean that these skills cannot be acquired. Many individuals find that the tasks and skills associated with online learning are easily mastered once appropriate instruction has been received. The following tips can also assist in helping you to successfully adapt and flourish in the online classroom.

Tip No. 1: Update Your Computer

Prior to enrolling in an online course of study, you must find out the computer requirements of your online school. Some of the most popular computer programs used in online learning include Microsoft Word, PowerPoint, and Adobe Acrobat Reader, and a common computer tool is Microsoft Excel, which is used to create and format spreadsheets. Once you find out the computer requirements, check your computer to see if these programs are already installed on your hard drive. Many computers already have these programs installed. For instance, if you purchased a computer that had Microsoft Office Suite installed on the hard drive, Microsoft Office Word, Microsoft Office Excel, and Microsoft Office PowerPoint are readily available for your use. Bear in mind, however, that these programs are updated from time to time, so it is wise to ask your online institution which version of certain software programs they require you to have. For example, students who have the 2003 version of Word may have a difficult time in opening documents sent to them from computer users who have the 2007 version of Word.

If you do not have a relatively new computer and you are planning on installing these programs into your computer, be sure there is sufficient memory on the hard drive so the programs can run correctly. Before purchasing software, check with the school because many schools provide software to the students at little or no charge. It is also possible to find programs such as Adobe Acrobat Reader online for free. If you will be purchasing a new computer, it is always a good idea to check with your online school to ensure that the model you purchase has the required software and is compatible with your online program. For example, one school strongly suggested that a student who already had a Macintosh computer purchase a Windows computer prior to the start of his coursework.

The important message here is that you should ensure you have the correct software on your computer for your courses and that your version of the program is compatible with that of your online institution. Most online universities offer information technology (IT) assistance to lend a hand to students in evaluating their computer needs and to help with program installation. Do not be afraid to ask for assistance. Remember, the online institution wants its students to succeed, so take advantage of their technology assistance. The small amount of time invested in making sure your computer programs are up to date and compatible with those of your online institution will definitely pay off.

Tip No. 2: Identify and Address Potential Internet Issues Early On

Problems can occur with insufficient Internet bandwidth (Pullen, 2006). Bandwidth can be compared to an underground pipeline. The size of the pipeline determines the amount of information that can travel at one time and the speed at which the information can travel. The larger the pipeline is, the greater the amount of information can travel through it and at a greater speed. Cable, DSL (digital subscriber line), and fiber optic access have a higher amount of bandwidth while dial-up access has a smaller amount of bandwidth. Dial-up access, therefore, is much slower and is limited in the amount of information that can travel through it at one time. This is one of the reasons that students find dial-up connections to be very frustrating. Most schools strongly recommend that you *do not* attempt to complete online classes with a dial-up connection to the Internet. The recommendation is to subscribe to a communication system that offers a higher amount of bandwidth, if possible.

Problems can also occur if the Internet provider that you are using frequently loses Internet connectivity. Being booted out of the classroom because of an unreliable Internet service provider can create a great deal of frustration and angst for the student being booted, the instructor, and the other students in the classroom who are communicating with each other. The best way to be prepared for Internet issues is to subscribe to a reliable Internet provider service. This is money well spent for online students!

Here are some additional tips to assist in dealing with Internet issues:

- Learn when public libraries are open and what their computer use policies are.
- If your home Internet service is inoperable, you may want to go to an Internet café for access, if you own a laptop.
- If the Internet service presents problems on a regular basis, you might want to consider changing Internet providers.
- Another option for problematic Internet service is to purchase an air card or mobile modem, which can provide access to the Internet wherever there is cell phone reception.
- If there is a group project when the Internet is inaccessible, you should have the telephone numbers of all of the group members readily available so you can phone them as needed until the Internet service is up and running.

Tip No. 3: Locate a Local Tech Support Person

It is recommended that you find a knowledgeable friend or family member who would be willing to act as a resource person if help is needed. When you are seeking out a local resource, look for someone who has good computer skills, who understands how to use the various software programs, and who can be readily available to assist in troubleshooting computer problems. While online programs do offer IT support, they may not be available quickly enough to assist in fixing the problem or the support person may not fully understand the problem that a student is trying to convey over the phone. Many students have found a local tech support person has been an invaluable resource to troubleshoot on the spot, particularly when there are time constraints and when a student is not really sure how to describe the problem.

Tip No. 4: Complete the Orientation Tutorial

It is crucial, and sometimes required, that students complete the online orientation tutorial offered by the school. The orientation tutorial can assist in helping students to become familiar with the program so that their energy may be expended on learning as opposed to struggling with the technical aspect of the program. Since many orientation tutorials contain practice opportunities in skills such as adding attachments to email, downloading and uploading documents or files, and developing a document, it gives students the opportunity to become familiar with the expectations of the program, and this can assist in minimizing anxiety, particularly for a technologically challenged student.

Tip No. 5: Understand How to Access Your Web-Based Classrooms

WebCT, Blackboard, E-College, and Angel are all examples of Web-based classrooms used in the online learning environment (Holly et al., 2008). Classrooms such as these enable schools to offer courses online in either a synchronous or asynchronous format. Synchronous communication occurs when all parties are present at the same time in the classroom or chat room. Asynchronous communication, however, does not require all parties to be present at the same time. Communication evolves over time as students and faculty respond to information that has been posted in the classroom or the chat room.

Online classrooms and scholastic chat rooms function in much the same manner as any online chat room. The students are required to (1) understand where to go to find the classroom or the chat room; (2) understand how to enter or sign in to the classroom or the chat room; and (3) understand how to participate in the classroom or chat room discussion. This information is usually clearly described in the course syllabus and/or classroom home page. Learn how to navigate your Web-based syllabus and classroom home page in order to find this information. Practice entering the classroom and also practice logging out of the classroom. These skills are not difficult to learn; they are simply different, and most students are amazed at how quickly they pick up on the process!

How to Minimize Bumps in the Road to Enhance the Learning Environment

Beginning a new course online holds similar issues as those faced in the traditional classroom setting. Most students realize that instructor preferences can vary widely and their preferences can affect assignments, tests, and even how the course itself is actually conducted. Since the online classroom does not provide the benefit of meeting with the instructor on a face-to-face basis, it is in your best interest to familiarize yourself with certain aspects of the online course prior to the actual start of the class in order to avoid potential frustration and anxiety.

Contacting the Course Instructor

Students will find that methods for contacting the course instructor along with times for contacting the instructor will vary. Some instructors will share their professional email address, personal email address, office phone number, and personal phone number, or any combination of the above. Others may only offer a professional email address and a phone number. As far as when to contact instructors, some instructors will be open to communication from students both day and night, while others post office hours and are only available during those times. Knowing how and when to contact the course instructor will help to minimize anxiety and frustration for both you and the instructor when questions and concerns arise.

Locating Support Service Information

It is important to know that online institutions offer various support services for their students. Support services generally include the library, course advisors, registrar, and technology support (also known as tech support or IT services). The link to these services may be listed on a variety of home pages, such as the course home page and the institution's home page. Be sure to perform a full review of the institution's Web site and familiarize yourself with the process of getting in touch with these specialty support services. You should also have this information hard copied and in an accessible location so it is readily available should any issues arise or if any information is needed. In addition, have on hand the hours of operation and the physical location of these services. It may be, for example, that the advisors are in California and the school library is in Kansas. You would then need to determine when to call for assistance based on the time zones. If assistance is offered, be sure to write down what the support personnel suggested for you to do. While you may think that you will remember what was suggested, it is extremely easy to forget the directions when under pressure. Having notes will save time and prevent further aggravation.

> **Tip**
>
> Print out a hard copy of the support service information and, if possible, have it laminated and sit it near your work space so the information is readily accessible and protected from accidental spills.

Assignments

Assignments in online programs are required in a variety of manners. Typically, assignments require that the students answer preassigned questions and then post a written response to the questions (Lorenzetti, 2005). These assignments can occur in either a live chat room (Christianson, Tiene, & Luft, 2002) or in the form of a discussion board. In a live chat room, assignments are often completed in a synchronous format where the students and the instructor are online at the same time. All parties discuss the answers together, enabling the students to learn from each other. Assignments completed in an asynchronous format generally occur on a discussion board. In this format, students and the instructor are not in the classroom at the same time, but instead read and respond to assignments that are posted in one central location. This type of assignment selection is based on the constructivism and adult learning theories (Holly et al., 2008; Wambach et al., 1999), which provides students a unique opportunity to learn from each other. These types of assignments have also been thought to improve written communication skills because they require responses that are thorough and thought provoking (Lorenzetti, 2005).

If you are asked to complete an assignment using a program or a format that is unfamiliar to you, budget additional time to complete it. For example, if you have never created a PowerPoint presentation or you have never worked on a data spreadsheet in Excel, start working on the assignment much earlier than the due date. While gathering information for the task may not take any additional time, presenting the information in the correct format is likely to be time consuming.

Similarities Between Online and Traditional Learning Programs

Traditional and online courses are surprisingly similar (Singh & Pan, 2004). Students are required to complete readings and demonstrate their understanding of various concepts through assignments. Students are also responsible for learning, actively participating in the class, and accessing research through Web-based databases.

Importance of Deadlines

The importance of meeting deadlines cannot be emphasized too strongly. Students, at times, become lackadaisical and do not submit work on time. Unfortunately, one of my students had to repeat a course because she lost so many points for submitting late assignments. Sometimes she did not turn anything in at all. This was a travesty because when she did submit her assignments they were superb and demonstrated that she was mastering the material.

Responsibility for Learning

Programs of higher education have moved from a teacher-centered to a learner-focused format (Holly et al., 2008), meaning that the teacher is no longer the center of the educational experience (Weimer, 2002). Learning is accomplished when students and the instructor collaborate, using life experiences to integrate previous knowledge with new knowledge, and making this new knowledge relevant to the students' individual situations or individual needs (Knowles, Holton, & Swanson, 2005).

In online courses, learners determine when to complete their assignments according to specific parameters and specific due dates (Wambach et al., 1999). While there is autonomy on the learner's part, it is still important to be aware of due dates and to submit assignments in a timely fashion. Instructors often post a schedule of assignments and due dates on the home page of the course. It is suggested that you print the schedule at the beginning of the course and use it to plan and manage your time effectively.

Active Participation

Participation in learning activities is required in both traditional and online learning formats. In the online format, however, a student's overall grade is affected by the quality of the written content submitted in the classroom along with the number of times the student participates in the classroom. In the online environment, each and every student is required to be an active participant, and it is this level of interaction between the students and the instructor that greatly enhances learning (Holly et al., 2008; Knowles et al., 2005; Lorenzetti, 2005; Singh & Pan, 2004).

Accessing Research Through Web-Based Databases

Students may access information for assignments through a traditional on-site library; however, it is common for information to be accessed through databases that are available in a virtual library. Both traditional and online programs can subscribe to the databases of their choice, thereby providing students access to scholarly journals that can be utilized to research information.

Identify which databases are available to you, or which databases are approved by your learning institution, and practice searching those databases in order to discover the journals available within each. Some databases will only provide abstracts, while others will provide complete articles. It is important that you become very comfortable using the databases in order to save precious time when searching for information. Examples of databases frequently used by nursing students are ProQuest Nursing & Allied Health Source, Ovid, and CINAHL; however, each discipline will find databases that are particularly useful when researching up-to-date information.

Common Myths About Online Education

There are two common myths about online education, which are: (1) this form of education is not as good as a traditional education, and (2) less work is required of the students. Singh and Pan (2004) discovered that educators found the online format to be of equal or better quality than the traditional classroom, with the end result being that the students had richer learning experiences.

Myth No. 1: Online Education Is Not as Good as Traditional Education

Arguments against the myth that online education is not as good as traditional education include studies, observations, and expert opinions.

- Pullen (2006) interviewed multiple students of online courses who believed that they experienced a superior level of learning in the online format, and that they actually received higher test scores than they had in traditional courses. These students stated that their grasp of the course material increased, and that the knowledge they gained was more relevant to their professional practice. They also shared that, overall, this format produced learning of a higher caliber.
- Wambach et al. (1999) found that students evaluated online courses positively overall. In addition, faculty members reported that the online discussions were insightful, and the writing quality of submitted assignments was equal to the quality of that submitted by traditional students.
- Assignments, such as threaded discussion questions, generally encourage more complex and critical thinking, as they require explanation and discourse among students (Wambach et al., 1999).
- When students are required to write responses to questions, communicate information, and express or defend opinions, an in-depth thought process and study of the material are necessities.
- When the students provide feedback to one another, additional thought-provoking questions are often presented that require further research that provides an opportunity for the students to consider, and possibly gain, a different perspective (Holly et al., 2008).
- When the learner takes responsibility for gaining information that is personally relevant, he or she takes personal ownership of the education (Holly et al., 2008).
- When students in online programs interact with their peers, they tend to solve problems on a higher plane of learning than that of their actual developmental level.
- When discussion occurs, the students gain deeper insight of the learning material, improve problem-solving skills, and develop critical thinking skills.

Myth No. 2: The Workload in Online Programs Is Lighter Than in Traditional Programs

The idea that there is less work required in an online course of study is another common myth. Certain online instructors express belief that students in online classes actually work harder and learn more than students in the traditional setting (Christianson et al., 2002; Ryan et al., 2004). Christianson and colleagues conducted a study involving online learners and their perspectives of student workload. One particular student in this study stated that in his opinion, the students in the online classroom actually work harder than students in a traditional classroom setting. He further explained that, in his experience, the students in online programs also demonstrated deeper insight and gained more knowledge of the material than students in traditional programs.

The reason for this could be explained by the types of questions used in online discussions, which often include comparing and contrasting, explaining opinions and positions on topics, reflective thinking, and examining the different perspectives of various issues (Holly et al., 2008). This type of questioning requires a greater effort and time commitment on the part of the students along with more complex reasoning than the true/false and multiple-choice questions that are often asked on traditional tests.

Conclusion

It is definitely possible for a technopeasant to successfully complete an online education program. A student who has basic computer skills and the required software and Internet accessibility should be able to learn the skills necessary to complete the program. Online programs provide students with the opportunity to access education, even if they would not otherwise be able to complete a traditional course of study. Online programs are even convenient for those who are busy with families, jobs, or other commitments. Students must understand that online programs are as effective as traditional programs and that they do require just as much work, if not more. It will be much less frustrating for students if plans are made to allow sufficient time to complete assignments, and, if problems should arise, alternate plans are made to resolve them. The best of luck to you with your online educational journey!

Checklist for Success

_______ Familiarize yourself with basic computer skills such as sending and receiving email, downloading and uploading documents, and searching the Web.

_______ Update your computer so that it meets the software requirements for the coursework.

_______ Identify and address potential Internet issues before class begins.

_______ Locate a local tech support person.

_______ Complete the online orientation tutorial offered by the school.

_______ Understand how to access and practice accessing your online classroom.

_______ Know how and when to contact the course instructor and support service personnel.

_______ Allow sufficient time to complete assignments.

_______ Plan for computer glitches.

_______ Print out class schedules, assignment due dates, and key phone numbers.

_______ Practice using the online databases to search for information and identify other useful online resources.

_______ Practice searching the Web for tutorials and other information.

_______ Become familiar with the software programs that are new to you.

_______ Enjoy the online learning experience and complete the course.

References

Christianson, L., Tiene, D., & Luft, P. (2002). Web-based teaching in undergraduate nursing programs [Electronic version]. *Nurse Educator,* 27(6), 276–282.

Holly, C., Legg, T. J., Mueller, D., & Adelman, D. S. (2008). Online teaching: Challenges for a new faculty role. *Journal of Professional Nursing, 24*(4), 254–258.

Knowles, M. S., Holton III, E. F., & Swanson, R. A. (2005). *The adult learner: The definitive classic in adult education and human resource development* (6th ed.). Boston: Elsevier.

Lorenzetti, J. P. (2005). Beyond multiple choice: Assessment for online learning. *Distance Education Report, 9*(18), 1, 6–7. Retrieved February 11, 2007 from EBSCOHost-ASP database.

Pullen, D. L. (2006). An evaluative case study of online learning for healthcare professionals [Electronic version]. *The Journal of Continuing Education in Nursing, 37*(5), 225–232.

Ryan, M., Carlton, K. H., & Ali, N. S. (2004). Reflections on the role of faculty in distance learning and changing pedagogies [Electronic version]. *Nursing Education Perspectives, 25*(2), 73–80.

Singh, P., & Pan, W. (2004). Online education: Lessons for administrators and instructors [Electronic version]. *College Student Journal, 38*(2), 302–308.

Wambach, K., Boyle, D., Hagemaster, J., Teel, C., Langner, B., Fazzone, P., et al. (1999). Beyond correspondence, video conferencing, and voice mail: Internet-based master's degree courses in nursing [Electronic version]. *Journal of Nursing Education, 38*(6), 267–271.

Weimer, M. (2002). *Learner-centered teaching: Five key changes to practice.* San Francisco: Jossey-Bass.

Chapter 2

How Do I Learn? Let Me Count the Ways: Learning Styles and Strategies

Patricia Clayburn

As the online learning environment becomes increasingly popular, discussion regarding individualized learning styles and strategies for the diverse online learner population gains importance. Research abounds on learning styles and multiple intelligences (Gardner, 1999). The relevance of these learning styles to the online course of study becomes more apparent than in the traditional classroom arena. In the online environment, greater emphasis is placed on the online adult learner being a self-starter, in control of his or her learning environment, and employing active learning strategies that result in the enhancement of that learning (Phillips, 2005).

This chapter identifies the learning styles that are most common among students, explains how to determine your own learning style, and details strategies that you can employ in order to succeed in the online environment. Whether you are a visual learner who benefits from seeing pictures and words, or a kinesthetic learner who needs more hands-on experiences, this chapter will present many tips to help you make the most of your online learning experience.

Overview of Theory

Investigation into individual learning styles is not a new phenomenon. The process of identifying different styles of learning is backed by over 30 years of research, which suggests that learners who are taught by methods corresponding to their preferred learning styles tend to apply the learning more effectively, retain the information for a longer period of time, and view their learning in a positive light (Moallem, 2007). There is a wealth of literature, theories, and models that assist in determining a student's preferred learning style, but, for the sake of brevity, we will highlight only a few in this chapter.

Learning Theory

Gardner's multiple intelligence theory suggests that all persons possess the following eight different intelligences: verbal-linguistic, logical-mathematical, visual-spatial, bodily-kinesthetic, rhythmic-musical, interpersonal, intrapersonal, and naturalistic. According to Gardner (1983), these intelligences complement and work with one another in the learning environment.

Chickering and Gamson (1987), utilizing a different perspective on learning, integrate the multiple intelligence theory as a framework for their principle of reciprocity and cooperation among students, which, briefly explained, is learning through collaboration with and in relation to others (Schrand, 2008).

Learning Models

Various learning style models have been developed over the past 30 years, including Kolb's learning styles, the Dunn and Dunn learning styles inventory, and the Felder-Silverman dimensions of learning style model.

Kolb's Learning Style Model

Kolb's learning style model arose from John Dewey's experiential learning theory. Dewey's experiential learning theory brought forth the concept that there is a relationship between learning and experience. Using Dewey's ideas, Kolb described learning as cyclical and occurring in stages, with new learning coming from new experiences (Bradshaw, 2004). In his model, Kolb identified the following four basic learning styles (Kolb, 1984):

1. Converger—prefers abstract conceptualization and active experimentation.
2. Diverger—prefers concrete conceptualization and reflective observation.
3. Assimilator—prefers abstract conceptualization and reflective observation.
4. Accommodator—prefers concrete experience and active experimentation.

Dunn and Dunn Learning Styles Inventory

The Dunn and Dunn learning styles inventory uses five categories, or elements, to help an individual determine how he or she prefers to learn. These five categories include environmental, emotional, sociological, physical, and psychological elements (Dunn & Dunn, 1978; Kitchie, 2003).

Felder-Silverman Dimensions of Learning Style Model

The Felder-Silverman model poses the following five fundamental questions to assist in identifying a student's style of learning:

1. What type of information does the student preferentially perceive?
2. Through what modality is sensory information most effectively perceived?
3. With which method of organization of information is the student most comfortable?
4. How does the student prefer to process information?
5. How does the student progress toward understanding?

These questions direct responses into the following five categories of learners: sensing, visual, inductive, active, and sequential (Felder & Silverman, 1988). The five questions in the Felder-Silverman model combined with the eight categories of Gardner's multiple intelligences theory can assist in not only identifying a student's style of learning but also in identifying the way he or she perceives and processes information.

Narrowing the Focus

Many of us intuitively know how we learn best. We have all made non-research-based comments about ourselves revealing our learning styles, such as, "I'm too antsy to sit still during a lecture," "I have to have pictures to look at," "I like to listen to audio lectures rather than sit in a classroom," "I read a whole chapter and I don't remember anything I've read," and "I learn best when I can interact with other people." These are all comments you are likely to have heard from friends and colleagues as well. Using the knowledge you already possess about your own preferred learning style is key in determining what methods are most effective for you.

As it would be a huge task to take every different learning inventory and pull the information together to identify your learning style, we shall narrow the focus of the remainder of this chapter to the following three well-known types of learners: visual, auditory, and kinesthetic.

Exploring Your Style

Although you probably have a good idea of what your learning style is, there are numerous books, articles, and Web sites that can help you to determine your learning style with a short test. By typing "learning style inventory" into a search engine, you can easily find many Web sites devoted to the topic. Be cautious, however, as some Web sites will charge for the results of these tests, while you can find the same information for free at other sites. At the time of this writing, two free and easy-to-use sites are http://www.personal.psu.edu/bxb11/LSI/LSI.htm and http://www.metamath.com/lsweb/dvclearn.htm.

Learning Styles and Strategies

Visual

The visual learner learns best by seeing. Colors, pictures, and visualization are all important to those who learn best by this method. Here are some strategies for the visual learner:

- Look at all of the study materials available (books, film, notes, etc.) and remember that some online programs include visual aid materials (DVDs, etc.) along with textbooks. Visual learners generally benefit from doing all of the assigned readings as well as searching out other visually stimulating sources that supplement the course material.

Creative Highlighting

One adult learner in a master's degree program utilized this strategy extremely effectively. Every week during the online discussion group, one main topic was explored by each student and then discussed with peers. This learner noted the main themes of each student's posting by writing notes about it and highlighting each theme with a different colored highlighter. She could later "see" those colors in her head, and associated each color with the theme it represented. This made it much easier to develop a paper on the subjects later.

- During a traditional classroom lecture, you can visualize pictures that correspond with the material presented orally by the instructor. Additionally, whether you are a student of either traditional or online programs, you can use different colors of pens and/or highlighters to take notes or to assist in identifying different themes or subjects that occur in the lectures or in the readings.
- If you need to see a concept, try mapping it out, as this enhances your ability to determine relationships and make connections (Bradshaw, 2004). Examples of and uses for concept mapping can be found easily by doing a search on the Web and in Figure 2-1.

FIGURE 2-1 Example of a Simple Concept Map

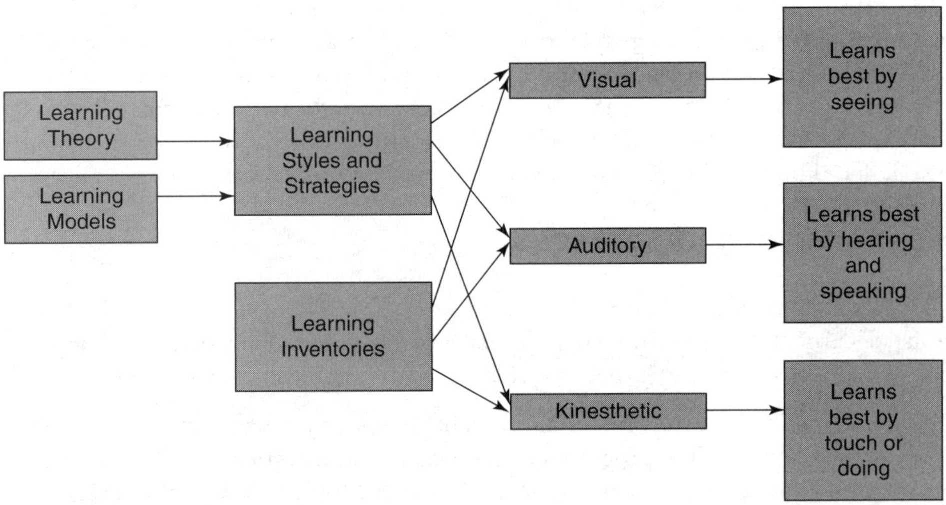

- When attempting to learn a new concept, close your eyes and visualize something connected to that concept. If you are a visual learner, this should help you to reinforce new concepts and ideas and it allows for easier mental retrieval later on.
- Review flash cards outlining important concepts.

Auditory

The auditory learner learns best by hearing and speaking. For these learners, simply reading the required reading can be frustrating, as they learn best by hearing the material and interacting with others through discussion. The online learning environment may be especially challenging for auditory learners, since so much of the time spent learning online is through reading. Online discussion groups, where peers post their work and then discuss the work with the class as a whole through written postings, can be overwhelming. Here are some strategies you can employ if you are an auditory learner:

- When reading through discussion postings, read them aloud to yourself. Summarize the important points and teach them out loud to someone else or yourself—yes, even if you are alone.
- Record yourself reading the assigned readings. You can use an iPod or MP3 player to listen to the recordings in the car or at any convenient time. This is like having an audio lecture.
- Take advantage of any audio lectures your professor may post online.
- If you are taking classes with a local group (from your place of employment, for example), plan frequent get-togethers to discuss the topics, to get feedback from each other, and to ask questions about the readings. Otherwise, ask if any of your online classmates would be interested in a study group that would entail phone or conference call communication.
- Be cautious about using background noise, such as music or television, when studying or doing coursework. Auditory learners are drawn to sounds, so this may actually make it more difficult for you to focus on the task at hand.

Some studies have found that one of the most important facets of online education is

Enlist Help!

I am an auditory learner. Requirements of my online master's degree program included posting to and participating in the discussion boards at least three times a week. All of that reading, in addition to the books and articles we also needed to read, was overwhelming to me at times. I began printing out the discussion threads and asking my husband to read them out loud to me. If he was unavailable, I would print them out and read them aloud to myself. You could also enlist a friend or other relative to assist with the reading process if this method appeals to you.

interaction with the instructors (Thiele, 2003). As an auditory learner who may be longing for verbal interaction, you will want to have your professor's contact information and find out how he or she prefers to be contacted. Although correspondence is typically done through email, most professors also have office hours during which they can be contacted for verbal feedback, either in person or by phone.

Don't Be Afraid to Ask!

A former colleague of mine confided in me a secret to his success while obtaining his bachelor's degree online. As an auditory learner, he missed receiving verbal feedback and instruction from professors. So, he contacted each instructor by email at the beginning of every course to ask if he could set up a weekly time where he would call that professor. He and the instructor would set up a short time (generally ten minutes long) each week where they could discuss any assignments and the professor could provide verbal instructions and/or feedback. My colleague feels this helped him tremendously through all of his courses, and he never had a professor refuse his request.

Kinesthetic

If you have ever said, "Don't tell me how to do something; show me, and then let me do it myself," then you are most likely a kinesthetic, or a hands-on type of learner. We mentioned earlier that auditory learners sometimes struggle in the online environment, and kinesthetic learners may as well. These types of learners typically learn best by touching or doing, making learning in the online environment a challenge. Here are some strategies that may help:

- Take frequent breaks when reading, writing, or engaging in online discussion groups. Kinesthetic learners often feel the need to move around frequently, and can become frustrated by inactivity and focusing on one thing for too long a period of time.
- When studying in short blocks of time, as mentioned previously, be active during your breaks. Move around, stretch, move to a different location for a few minutes, etc.
- Do something tactile. Hold a pen or a hot or cold drink in your hand(s) when you are studying or reading course material or take notes as you read and participate in the discussion forums.

Take a Breather!

One of my peers in my online master's degree program was a kinesthetic learner and was frustrated at first by sitting at the computer for long periods of time. She solved this problem with creative scheduling and a timer. She wrote out a very specific schedule for her times at the computer: no more than 30 minutes at a time, then a 15-minute break. During the break, she sometimes went outdoors or just did something tactile indoors, such as working on a craft project. Knowing that she would be sitting at the computer for no more than 30 minutes also helped to keep focused on the material.

- Use a small, portable fan to help experience the sense of touch or feel while learning.
- Walk while reading or studying. (Warning: Do not try this while walking on stairs or in traffic!) Chewing gum or snacking on something light and healthy can also help.
- Draw a sketch of an idea you are studying. Some kinesthetic learners have even built models of concepts, enabling them to incorporate doing into the learning process.

Conclusion

Every individual learns differently. Whether you are a visual, auditory, or kinesthetic learner (or if you fall into one of any number of other categories), there are ways to make the online learning environment work for you. Be creative and search out your own strategies to aid in your individualized learning. Be sure to continue to evaluate your progress and learning on an ongoing basis, in order to make any adjustments needed for your own style. Take a personal inventory every few weeks by asking yourself if you are grasping concepts well, if you are engaged in the learning process, and if you are enjoying the class or program. By assessing your individual learning style and utilizing some of the strategies mentioned in this chapter, you will make your online learning experience personalized, fun, and rewarding!

Overall Checklist for Learning Style Strategies

_______ Familiarize yourself with learning style concepts by reading this chapter.

_______ Take a learning style inventory online at:
http://www.personal.psu.edu/bxb11/LSI/LSI.htm or
http://www.metamath.com/lsweb/dvclearn.htm, or through another venue.

_______ Read through the tips and strategies in this chapter that apply to your determined learning style.

_______ Begin to use the individualized strategies listed in this chapter (see the specific learning style checklists that follow).

_______ Create your own personalized strategies.

_______ Evaluate your progress on a regular basis to ascertain which strategies are working and which may not be.

Checklist for the Visual Learner

_______ Familiarize yourself with the basic concepts of visual learning in this chapter.

_______ Make use of all the study materials available to you, including books and other visual aid materials such as DVDs.

_______ Visualize something connected to the concepts as you read for easier mental retrieval later.

_______ Use colored highlighters to highlight different themes or subjects that occur in your readings.

_______ Try concept mapping (see Figure 2-1).

_______ Try using flash cards to outline concepts when reviewing coursework.

Checklist for the Auditory Learner

_______ Familiarize yourself with the basic concepts of auditory learning in this chapter.

_______ Read discussion postings in the online classroom out loud to yourself or enlist help from family or friends in reading them out loud to you.

_______ Record yourself reading the assigned readings using an iPod or MP3 player to listen to when convenient.

_______ Listen to any audio lectures posted by the professor.

_______ Be careful of background noise when studying, as it can be very distracting to auditory learners.

_______ Form a local study group to meet and discuss the topics.

_______ Form an online study group to meet, via phone or conference call, to discuss the topics.

_______ Keep in touch with the professor via phone to receive verbal feedback.

Checklist for the Kinesthetic Learner

_______ Familiarize yourself with the concepts of kinesthetic learning in this chapter.

_______ Take frequent breaks when reading or when participating in online discussion boards.

_______ Be active during those breaks.

_______ Do something tactile while studying. Take notes or hold something in your hands.

_______ Use a small fan to help you experience the sense of feel while learning.

_______ Walk, chew gum, or snack on something light while reading or studying. (Warning: Do not try this while walking on stairs or in traffic!)

_______ Draw a sketch of an idea or a concept you are studying.

References

Bradshaw, M. J. (2004). Effective learning: What teachers need to know. In A. J. Lowenstein & M. J. Bradley (Eds.), *Fuszard's innovative strategies in nursing* (3rd ed., pp. 3–17). Sudbury, MA: Jones and Bartlett.

Chickering, A., & Gamson, Z. (1987). Seven principles of good practice in undergraduate education. *American Association for Health Education Bulletin, 39*(7), 3–6.

Dunn, R., & Dunn, K. (1978). *Teaching students through their individual learning style.* Upper Saddle River, NJ: Prentice Hall.

Felder, R. M., & Silverman, L. (1988). Learning and teaching styles in engineering education. *Engineering Education, 78*(7), 674–681.

Gardner, H. (1983). *Frames of mind: The theory of multiple intelligences.* New York: Basic Books.

Gardner, H. (1999). *Intelligence reframed: Multiple intelligences for the 21st century.* New York: Basic Books.

Kitchie, S. (2003). Determinants of learning. In S. B. Bastable (Ed.), *Nurse as educator: Principles of teaching and learning for nursing practice* (2nd ed., pp. 75–118). Sudbury, MA: Jones and Bartlett.

Kolb, D. A. (1984). *Experiential learning: Experience as the source of learning and development.* Upper Saddle River, NJ: Prentice Hall.

Moallem, M. (2007). Accommodating individual differences in the design of online learning environments: A comparative study. *Journal of Research on Technology in Education, 40*(2), 217–245.

Phillips, J. S. (2005). Strategies for active learning in online continuing education. *The Journal of Continuing Education in Nursing, 36*(2), 77–83.

Schrand, T. (2008). Tapping into active learning and multiple intelligences with interactive multimedia: A low-threshold classroom approach. *College Teaching, 56*(2), 78–84.

Thiele, J. E. (2003). Learning patterns of online students. *Journal of Nursing Education, 42*(8), 364–366.

Chapter 3

Strategies to Deal with Expected Challenges

Stacia Thompson

The online learning environment requires a great deal of time, energy, motivation, diligence, and hard work (Hopper, 2007). Integrating online educational goals with work and family schedules takes discipline and patience, even in the most ideal situations. However well prepared a student may feel upon entering the online scholastic environment, challenges still may emerge that require that student to reevaluate his or her personal and academic goals. While certain challenges can be circumvented with advance planning, others require flexibility and creativity in order to maintain one's focus on meeting educational goals. This chapter offers strategies to plan for challenges that can exist before the coursework starts, as well as those that can arise afterwards.

Strategies

Obstacles such as work, age, family responsibilities, learning disabilities, military deployment, language barriers, and taking multiple courses at the same time are some adversities that can exist before coursework ever starts. Unfortunately, expected challenges such as these can deter a learner from fully engaging in coursework or achieving academic goals. Strategies that can be used to address these issues include the following: communication, management of time, delegation, celebration, assessment of Internet status and proficiency, and disclosure of learning disabilities.

Communication

Family Communication

Engaging family members in your online plan of study before starting coursework helps to foster teamwork and strategic planning, thereby initiating family cooperation. Continued communication with your family throughout the course of the program provides support and encouragement, which are especially important when encroaching deadlines require your undivided attention. Provide your family with your assignment calendar so they are aware of your schedule and associated time requirements. Integrate family functions and daily schedules, such as soccer practice and music lessons, into this calendar. Ensure that everyone's needs are identified and addressed appropriately. In this fashion, you acknowledge that family time is important and that everyone plays a key role in achieving the desired goals. Advance planning makes everyone's life easier, while also teaching the family about prioritization and helping others to realize personal goals.

Employer Communication

Communicating your online education plans with your employer provides essential information to those you work with regarding your schedule and time requirements. In addition, talking with your supervisor and coworkers provides the opportunity to learn about any resources available to employees returning to the classroom. Furthermore, clarification regarding the expectations of your workplace may help to prevent problems that can arise during the course of your online program. For instance, your employer may not allow access to workplace computers for coursework. Establishing computer use guidelines prior to the start of your program will preclude potential conflicts with your supervisor and coworkers.

Remember that your supervisor and coworkers can provide much-needed support during your classroom experience. Keep them apprised of your progress, deadlines, and associated issues. Simple communication courtesies demonstrated in the workplace can mean the difference between successful integration of work and school as well as unnecessary frustration in both arenas.

Instructor Communication

Communication with instructors is crucial in the online environment. Online instructors are aware of the recurrent need for flexibility, as unexpected situations do often arise. Accommodations needed for special situations or circumstances should be communicated to the instructor in a prompt and explicit manner. Issues such as learning disabilities, language fluency, family emergencies, a natural disaster, or military deployment to a remote location require instructor awareness. The online instructor is able to accommodate a variety of special circumstances, provided that you are willing to communicate your needs in a courteous and timely manner.

Instructor Communication

A student at a community college was deployed to Iraq during her final semester in the associate degree nursing program. Through special arrangements, she was able to complete the theory portion of the program. When she returned to the United States, further arrangements were made for her to complete the clinical portion of the program so she could obtain her degree.

Do not hesitate to contact your instructor if questions or difficulties occur. The virtual classroom allows students to send messages whenever issues arise. Check your classroom home page for instructor dialogue directives and contact information. In addition, scan the home page, class bulletin boards, and syllabus to find the answers to frequently asked questions and to check for updated course information.

Classmate Communication

Classmates in the online environment represent a very diverse cross-section of cultures, professions, backgrounds, and ages, and all of these classmates provide rich resources of information and support. Becoming acquainted with other students who share similar interests and values can be your best source of support and encouragement. Networking with online classmates provides valuable perspectives, insights, and opportunities similar to those found in the traditional classroom. An additional benefit of connecting with your e-classmates is gaining the support of those who are experiencing comparable situations. According to Thomas (2007), working and sharing with others in similar circumstances can help you to feel less overwhelmed.

Language Barriers and Communication

Students with limited English proficiency may consider utilizing translation tools for their assignments because there is an array of online translation tools, resources, and software packages available for students (Chong & Farago, 2005). These tools can be used to find appropriate words to express oneself or to translate the words of the instructor or classmates to improve understanding. As helpful as these tools can be, it is extremely important to remember that words or phrases are not always translated into their intended meaning. All languages contain subtleties that are not easily translated and can be misunderstood. When someone is in doubt regarding the meaning of a word or phrase, the best solution is to ask for help.

The Master Chicks

As a graduate student in an online program, I became a part of a tightly knit group of women, and it all started with an online chat. Several of us met on a Sunday afternoon just to talk. We soon discovered that we had a lot more in common than just our nursing classes. Because of one super coordinator who was involved, we did become an organized group. We even came up with a name—the Master Chicks! We communicated regularly via email and phone throughout the program. When someone was down or frustrated, someone else was there to provide encouragement.

When we finally met at graduation (in our matching shirts), it was a truly momentous occasion! I credit the Master Chicks with my ability to complete the program with my sanity intact. We have continued our online relationship since graduation, and this group remains a valued part of my life to this day.

Language Barriers

In one of my online courses, I had an instructor from Saudi Arabia. It was obvious that English was not his native language. He was, however, perfectly capable of sharing his thoughts and providing excellent feedback on my assignments, as he did not hesitate to ask for clarification if my writing was not completely clear to him.

Management of Time

Time management is a very personal issue; no two students have identical needs or requirements of their time. Therefore, it is important to remember that while there are many effective resources designed to help you manage your time effectively, it is up to you to adapt your specific needs to any type of time management program. Planning ahead of time will help you to maintain control of your time (Ellis, 2006).

Sample Time Usage Evaluation

Keep track of what you do every day for a full week. Keep track of the entire day—including the hours you sleep!

Assess Current Use of Time

The first step in setting up a time management program is an assessment of your current time needs (Ellis, 2006). To do this, monitor your time allocations for 1 week. Write down how much time is spent daily on each and every activity. If you currently utilize a personal daily planner (PDA) for your schedule, this exercise can simply be a review of your weekly calendar.

After you have accumulated your weekly data, it is time to identify and organize activities into categories such as study time, car pool, family time, housekeeping, etc. This provides you with a clear snapshot of how your time is spent. Once this is accomplished, you are able to decide where changes should be made.

Set Priorities

Determine what activities are most important to you and your family, and place these items in a list in order of importance. Identify those activities that are essential and those that are not. If time is limited, identify activities that can be delegated or eliminated altogether. Make sure to include family members in the discussion.

Devise a Time Schedule

Begin by entering the activities that do not vary from day to day or week to week, such as work hours, sleep hours, mealtime, and time needed to prepare children for school (Ellis, 2006). Make every attempt to stay as close as possible to your current schedule to avoid confusion. Then, add your scheduled family time. Scheduling family time requires creativity and flexibility, particularly with older children who are involved in numerous activities. After family time is entered, be sure to include at least 2 hours a week for yourself. Personal time should include whatever you like, such as watching television, going on a date with your spouse, or taking a trip to the local spa.

The next step is to incorporate your class schedule. Include time for all related tasks such as reading, research, synchronous/asynchronous chats, and assignment preparation and development. Many students find it beneficial to utilize the same time each day for their studies. This develops a predictable routine for both these students and their families.

Schedule a time period where interruptions and distractions will be at a minimum. Be realistic, and add time for any special needs you may have. For example, learning-disabled

Assess Current Use of Time

Time	Activity
6:00 a.m.	Get ready for work
6:30	Wake up kids & get them ready for school
7:00	Breakfast
7:30	Carpool to school/work
8:00	Work
8:30	Work
9:00	Work
9:30	Work
10:00	Work
10:30	Work
11:00	Work
11:30	Work
12:00 p.m.	Work
12:30	Work
1:00	Work
1:30	Work
2:00	Work
2:30	Work
3:00	Carpool for school
4:00	Relax
4:30	Take kids to soccer practice/Work on my schoolwork during practice
5:00	Soccer practice/continue to work on my schoolwork
5:30	Home from soccer practice/start dinner
6:00	Fix dinner/start kids on homework assignments
6:30	Dinner
7:00	Help kids with homework
7:30	Homework con't
8:00	Free time
8:30	Free time
9:00	Kids to bed/work on schoolwork
9:30	Work on schoolwork
10:00	Bed!

students report that school work takes more time, effort, and self-discipline than those without learning disabilities (Heiman & Precel, 2003).

Allow time for the unforeseen. Remember, while schedules are valuable tools for developing time management skills, they should never be so rigid as to not allow for the unexpected. Expect to be flexible and that you will occasionally make mistakes (see Table 3–1).

Scheduling with Young Children

Students with young children at home may find it especially difficult to work around their children's ongoing needs. Young children, particularly those under elementary school age, require a great deal of parental supervision and guidance. This can make finding quality study time a difficult, though not impossible task.

Attempt to schedule playgroups with other children. The rotational basis of hosting a playgroup provides you with valuable alone time for your studies. Seek out other online students in your area with young children who are also in need of study time, or other parents who simply want to provide quality playtime for their children. Check with your neighborhood schools and churches to see if they sponsor a "parent's day out" program or other form of weekly supervised playtime. These special events not only provide you with needed and valuable study time, but afford your children the opportunity to make new friends and to develop social skills.

Scheduling with School-Age Children and Adolescents

Time and attention issues with school-age children and adolescents present a different set of challenges. Providing your children with attention when they first come home from school or from child care should be a consistent priority. This can be done by talking with them about their day and by reviewing plans for after-school and evening activities. This short time of focused attention will help all of you to connect with each other and then move on to the next activity (Ellis, 2006).

Another way to connect is to plan study time together. If you have a large dining room table, give each person a designated space and sit down to study together. Use a kitchen timer to remind you to take regular breaks to talk with your children about what they are learning and to share what you are learning. Parents who are students can be role models for their children, demonstrating that education is a lifelong process.

Ask Your Children to Help

- Having problems figuring out how to use the computer? Ask your children for help. The younger generation has been using computers ever since they started school. Computers do not intimidate them.
- Having trouble keeping to the schedule? Ask your children to help. They can keep you on track.
- Need help studying for a test? Ask your children to quiz you.

Older children are frequently more involved in extracurricular and social activities than younger children. If possible, plan to do your classroom work when your children are involved in these activities. Read assignments or look over notes while the team warms up before the game. Use a backpack, computer bag, or basket to carry all of your school essentials that may be needed while on the road. While managing a family, children, a work schedule, and a study schedule can be difficult, it can also be quite rewarding.

> **Pizza Night**
>
> My stepdaughter and her family have always worked hard to set aside family time in spite of their busy schedules. They have been having a family pizza night for at least 15 years! There are no specific plans except that the family all gets together to eat and enjoy being together. This has been so important to the whole family that even the college-aged daughter makes it a point to come as often as possible.

Display the Time Schedule

All family members should review the schedule upon completion for accuracy. Ensure that the schedule is realistic and achievable. Provide each family member with a copy of the schedule, or post one master schedule in a common area. Be sure to note the frustrations and successes of the schedule during the week. Build on what works and discard what does not. Work toward a schedule that fits your family's needs. A workable schedule assists in keeping everyone on track and in control of his or her time.

Use Unscheduled Time

Even with the majority of your time accounted for in your weekly schedule, small segments of unscheduled time should still exist. For instance, while waiting for your child after ball practice or before an appointment, you can read your next assignment. Always carry a book or article you need to read with you in order to take advantage of these opportune moments. If you use a laptop computer and have Internet connectivity, use this time to check your e-class Web site for new announcements or assignment submissions by your classmates. Having a to-do list on hand at all times can help to maximize the use of unscheduled time.

> **Sample To-Do List for School Activities**
>
> 1. Finish reading assignment.
> 2. Outline response for discussion question.
> 3. Find additional resources to support ideas.
> 4. Look at criteria for project due in 4 weeks.
> 5. Email project partner to divide work.
> 6. Check online for any announcements.
> 7. Check online discussion board; respond as needed.

Delegation

It can be said that when a parent goes back to school, the entire family goes back to school as well. Look upon entering the e-classroom environment as an opportunity for your family to grow and develop together. Dunham (2004) suggests that the entire family make a list of necessary daily and weekly chores that must be completed and then delegate specific tasks to specific individuals. You should only address things that absolutely must be done. Tasks or events that can wait until more time is available can be pushed to the side. For instance, older children who can drive or who can work safely in the kitchen can help with errands and meals. Spouses and children can assist with housekeeping, yard work, and laundry. Young children can assist as well by doing things such as dusting, feeding the pets, or picking up toys. Ensure that tasks are assigned in accordance with the family members' abilities. Do not expect perfection; rather, graciously accept everyone's contribution to the overall benefit of the family and celebrate accomplishments together.

Solving the Sock Dilemma

I had a colleague who delegated the laundry responsibilities to her husband when she went back to school. She knew that he would throw all of the socks in his drawer without sorting them, which really bothered her. She did not want people to see him wearing socks that did not match! Her simple solution was to buy him socks that were all exactly the same. That way, it did not matter that he threw all of the socks in the drawer and pulled out the two that were on top each day.

Celebration

Celebrating the completion of a project or a big writing assignment with your family can serve several purposes, including the following: (1) it encourages your family to share in your accomplishments; (2) it assists in keeping your family up to date with where you are in your course of your study; (3) it provides your family with an opportunity to see that each step is bringing you, and them, closer to the end of the course, the end of the program, or maybe even graduation. Celebration of personal accomplishments during school should not be underestimated because it can also serve to keep you motivated (Carter, 2009), particularly when you may feel that there is no light at the end of the tunnel.

Celebrate Your Accomplishments

- Post your grades on the refrigerator alongside those of your children.
- Plan special treats for the whole family as you complete milestones like your first class, the halfway point of the program, and especially graduation.
- Allow yourself to have some downtime. This is particularly important for students who have a hard time taking a break from their studies.

Assessing Internet Status and Computer Proficiency

Assessment of your current Internet status prior to starting any online program is essential. After all, your ability to access your online classroom depends upon your Internet service provider and the quality of the connection. Investigate the cost of obtaining the highest quality Internet service available in your area. Upgrading your current home connection is a wise investment in terms of time and avoided frustration. However, if personal or situational constraints do not allow for Internet upgrades, alternatives are available. Free Internet connection resources may be available at the public library, a local coffee shop, or, with approval, at your place of employment. Bear in mind that while these businesses may offer free access, they do not guarantee that study space will be available when you need it. Consider your options wisely before choosing, and weigh the ultimate costs of lower technology in terms of time, frustration, availability, and ease of access.

If you have little or no computer experience, consider taking a basic computer skills course prior to enrolling in your online degree program. Courses are available in many areas through the continuing education offerings of public schools, community colleges, and universities. Basic courses include computer skills such as keyboarding, sending an email, posting to a discussion board, and attaching a file to an email or drop box. Students in advanced courses commonly use programs such as Microsoft PowerPoint and Excel. Online degree programs assume that students enrolling in their programs have a basic working knowledge of computers. Refreshing or upgrading your computer skills will enhance your ability to function in the online environment and avoid certain frustration.

Disclosing Learning Disabilities

Having a learning disability does not preclude enrolling in an online course of study. Knowing yourself and your capacity to deal with your situation, possessing a high degree of determination, emotional stability, and the utilization of support services have all shown to be good predictors of success in education (Heiman & Precel, 2003).

The rights of students with learning disabilities are protected by federal law. Section 504 of the Rehabilitation Act of 1973 and the Americans with Disabilities Act (ADA) require that students in higher education be given equal access, and that reasonable accommodations be provided (Frank & Halstead, 2005; Westby, 2000). However, no clear guidelines exist as to what exactly constitutes reasonable accommodations.

According to Westby (2000), a learning-disabled student should disclose his or her specific disability and provide required documentation in order to receive necessary accommodations. Each institution provides accommodations according to its specific institutional guidelines and policies. Ultimately, however, the responsibility for obtaining accommodations rests with the student.

Ask who to contact during your registration process in order to procure special accommodations. Disclose all information related to your disability honestly and to the best of your ability. Likewise, provide the required documentation to support the diagnosis of your disability. Be certain that your scholastic institution documents your disability correctly because your ability to obtain accommodations may be dependent upon the exact description of your condition.

Once your learning disability is documented, you can dialogue with the institution regarding specific accommodations required in order for you to successfully participate in the online classroom. Accommodation guidelines for online courses are more ambiguous than those for the traditional classroom; therefore, it is vital that you know what special accommodations you require. For example, the University of Washington (2008) suggests that a student with a learning disability have a complete understanding of his or her specific disability and how it impacts his or her learning style. Approaching the online institution fully prepared and knowledgeable of your disability demonstrates to the institution your determination and motivation to participate in the online classroom environment.

Possible accommodations for online learning include course content available in audio or video formats, adjustments to communication guidelines for class participation, increased availability of technical support, and phone contact with course faculty (Banerjee, 2002). New advancements in technology, such as programs to convert text to speech and phonetic spell checkers, provide even greater opportunities for disabled students. Contact the representative for students with special needs or other designated individual at your online institution to discuss available options.

Conclusion

Online education is an excellent tool for many individuals to reenter the classroom environment. The flexibility, convenience, and relative ease of access of the online classroom lure students pursuing advanced degrees. However, just as in the traditional classroom, the online learning environment can present certain challenges for the learner. By evaluating personal situations and considering potential stumbling blocks, a student can effectively address these issues and continue toward his or her scholastic goals. Preparation, a realistic attitude, patience, and support are the tools that help students to navigate life situations that may arise over the course of the online journey.

TABLE 3-1 Sample Time Schedule

Day/Time	Sun	Mon	Tues	Wed	Thurs	Fri	Sat
6:00 a.m.		Get ready for work	Get ready for work	Get ready for work	Get ready for work	Get ready for work	
6:30		Drive to work	Drive to work	Drive to work	Drive to work	Drive to to work	
7:00		Work	Work	Work	Work	Work	
7:30		Work	Work	Work	Work	Work	
8:00	Church	Work	Work	Work	Work	Work	
8:30	Church	Work	Work	Work	Work	Work	
9:00	Church	Work	Work	Work	Work	Work	
9:30		Work	Work	Work	Work	Work	

Day/Time	Sun	Mon	Tues	Wed	Thurs	Fri	Sat
10:00		Work	Work	Work	Work	Work	
10:30 . . .		Work	Work	Work	Work	Work	
3:00 p.m.		Work	Work	Work	Work	Work	My time
3:30		Pick kids up	Pick kids up	Pick kids up	Pick kids up	Pick kids up	My time
4:00	School time	Kids delivered to activities	Kids delivered to activities	Kids delivered to activities	Kids delivered to activities	To park with kids	My time
4:30	School time	Online time	Online time	Online time	Online time	To park with kids	My time
5:00	School time	Online time	Online time	Online time	Online time	To park with kids	
5:30	School time	Fix supper	Fix supper	Fix supper	Fix supper	Family time—pizza and movie	
6:00		Supper	Supper	Supper	Supper	Family time	
6:30						Family time	
7:00						Family time	
7:30						Family time	
8:00	Kids to bed	Kids to bed	Kids to bed	Kids to bed	Kids to bed	Family time	Kids to bed
8:30		School time	School time	School time	School time	Family time	
9:00		School time	School time	School time	School time		
9:30		School time	School time	School time	School time		
10:00							
10:30	To bed	To bed	To bed	To bed	To bed	To bed	To bed

Checklist to Deal with Expected Challenges

______ Communicate throughout the program to minimize frustrations and potential conflicts.

- ______ Family
- ______ Employer
- ______ Instructor
- ______ Classmates

______ Manage time efficiently

- ______ Assess current use of time
- ______ Set priorities
- ______ Devise a time schedule
- ______ Schedule time with young children
- ______ Schedule time with school-age children and adolescents
- ______ Use unscheduled time

______ Delegate chores and tasks

______ Celebrate accomplishments

______ Assess Internet status and computer proficiency

______ Disclose learning disabilities

References

Banerjee, M. (2002). *Distance education and accommodations for students with learning disabilities: Implications for post secondary service providers.* Retrieved January 2, 2009, from http://www.resourceroom.net/older/distance_ed.asp

Carter, W. Y. (2009). *Finishing your degree: So close but still a ways to go: 10 techniques to help you finish your degree.* Retrieved July 7, 2009, from http://www.tadafinallyfinished.com/newsletter/2009/newsjan09B.htm

Chong, A., & Farago, C. (2005). Encouraging participation in the multicultural classroom: Using visual resources. In *On diversity in teaching and learning: A compendium* (pp. 33–37). Boulder: University of Colorado at Boulder. Retrieved January 16, 2009, from http://www.colorado.edu/ftep/downloads/ondiversity.pdf#page=38

Dunham, K. S. (2004). *How to survive and maybe even love nursing school: A guide for students by students* (2nd ed.). Philadelphia: F.A. Davis Company.

Ellis, D. (2006). *Becoming a master student* (11th ed.). Boston: Houghton Mifflin Company.

Frank, B., & Halstead, J. A. (2005). Teaching students with disabilities. In D. M. Billings & J. M. Halstead (Eds.), *Teaching in nursing: A guide for faculty* (2nd ed., pp. 67–84). St. Louis, MO: Elsevier Saunders.

Heiman, T., & Precel, K. (2003). Students with learning disabilities in higher education: Academic strategies profile. *Journal of Learning Disabilities, 36*(3), 248–258.

Hopper, C. H. (2007). *Practicing college: Learning strategies.* Boston: Houghton Mifflin Company.

Thomas, K. (2007). *Successful online learning: Tips for taking your first online class.* Retrieved December 29, 2008, from http://distance-education.suite101.com/article.cfm/successful_online_learning

University of Washington. (2008). *College survival skills: Tips for students with disabilities to increase college success.* Retrieved January 2, 2009, from http://washington.edu/doit/Brochures/Academics/survival.html

Westby, C. (2000). Who are adults with learning disabilities and what do we do about them? *Topics in Language Disorders, 21*(1), 1–14.

Chapter 4

Strategies to Deal with Unexpected Challenges

Deborah Schlief

A hurricane in Florida, a flash flood in Texas, or even the death of a loved one may be some of the unexpected challenges facing the online learner. Even the most organized student could find himself or herself falling behind or thinking about dropping a course when a crisis is added on top of the everyday responsibilities of work, family, and school. Let us examine some specific challenges and solutions in an effort to better prepare you, in the unfortunate event that any of these occurrences affects your life while enrolled in an online program.

Natural Disasters

Challenges with Hurricanes, Floods, or Other Storms

Dependence on electricity for completion and submission of online assignments presents one of the most common challenges when a hurricane, flood, or other storm disrupts the power supply. Although you may be prepared and complete your assignment in a timely manner, the lack of electricity might make it impossible to submit your assignments in a typical fashion. Or you may be fortunate enough to maintain power during a natural disaster, but your Internet connection could go down with no hope for connectivity to be restored in the near future.

We also depend on functional hardware and software to complete assignments and to conduct research for projects. During severe weather events, equipment may be damaged from rain, wind, rising water, or a crushing blow. Because personal safety must come first, it may be necessary to evacuate your area rapidly during the storm, leaving unprotected equipment behind. Bringing a laptop and flash drive to the evacuation destination may be a possibility, but if the storm is sudden or your equipment is not portable, evacuation presents a real challenge to completing and submitting online assignments.

Solutions to Challenges

Proper prioritization in a natural disaster is key. Once you and your family have completed preparations for safety during the storm or flood, attention can be directed to your computer equipment and your class requirements (Texas Woman's University, 2007b). If there is ample warning before a severe weather event strikes, locate resources within your community scheduled for power and Internet restoration immediately after the storm. Local libraries, colleges, or hospitals with community access to their computer equipment are frequently the first to have electrical services restored. Keep notes on these local resources secured along with your other school equipment so that it is readily available. This knowledge may prevent serious delays in submitting your assignments.

Communicate with fellow students and your instructor regarding your situation as soon as possible. Your classmates may have experienced a similar situation and might be able to provide you with useful ideas. Your instructor may make arrangements for you to turn in your assignment early or late, depending on how soon the weather is expected to affect your area. Remember, the prediction of a strike zone is variable, and storms may veer off course. It is always reasonable to prepare for the worst while hoping for the best. Advance preparation can save you much frustration in the event of a direct hit by a storm or flood.

Your computer equipment can be damaged by rain, rising water, and flying or falling debris. If time allows, move your equipment to an area that is unlikely to be damaged by the weather, such as your place of evacuation. If the equipment is to remain in the area of concern, double bag it with plastic, place it on a table or other high surface to protect it from rising water, and situate it in a corner or in a small, windowless room (Ferguson & Watson, 2003).

Gather all original software and paper items, such as reports and books, and place them in a rigid, watertight container. Back up all online documents on a travel or flash drive to store with your software, so that they are readily accessible after the storm. Prepare a list of items stored in the container and secure the list inside the container, on top of those items packed. After the storm is over, you may not remember what you stored where, and the list may prove invaluable to your recovery. If evacuation is necessary, it may also be helpful to prepare a list of what should go with you to the evacuation location. Space may be at a premium, both during the trip to your evacuation area and during your stay at the new location.

If you are located in an area that is prone to seasonal storms or floods, there is no need to wait for an impending disaster to make preparations. Just as residents living in hurricane zones prepare their storm kits with food and water on a yearly basis, a little advance preparation by the

Hit by a Hurricane

Before we were hit by a hurricane, I printed out my assignment for the week and tried to focus on completing as much of it as possible. I let my classmates and my instructor know ahead of time that we were expecting a direct hit and that I had no idea when power and Internet would be restored afterwards. I saved my discussions on my travel drive, as my instructor did not want me to post early, but she did say that I should post as soon as possible after the storm. I made notes and packed everything into a plastic bin. After the storm, we were without power for 5 days, and Internet access was restored at about the same time. There was so much to do afterwards, both for my family and for school, that I found it difficult to concentrate, but I did manage to submit my discussion on time and did not lose any points.

online student can save much time and grief. *Always* back up your work on a secure, portable device, such as a travel drive. You may want to consider storing your backups and your original software discs in an offsite location, such as a safe deposit box, if a tornado or fire strikes. You also may want to consider printing your syllabus and weekly assignments at the beginning of each class during storm season. Stay on schedule for your assignments or, better yet, work a week ahead if at all possible so that you are prepared in case a storm comes up suddenly. The purchase of a laptop computer may be the key to your peace of mind, as it is easily portable and can be used with battery power in the case of an electrical outage. However, this does still require diligence on your part to keep the battery fully charged.

Recovery Plan

After the storm or flood has passed and it is safe to return to home and normal activity, the online student can utilize any resource information obtained during the planning phase. Properly stored and protected equipment and class information can make this task as simple as unpacking your belongings. If power outages and disruption in Internet access continue, use your list of public resources, such as local libraries or hospital computer centers, to see if they are up and running. It may be possible to post your assignments and discussions at those locations until the situation is resolved at your home.

Continue to communicate with your classmates and instructor by phone until you are able to resume normal operations (Zsohar & Smith, 2008). Your instructor can help you to develop a recovery timeline for your assignments so that you are not penalized for a situation beyond your control.

Keep in mind the importance of taking care of yourself and your family. There is so much to do in the recovery phase after a natural disaster that it can be seriously overwhelming. Eventually things will return to normal, although a *new* normal may be the case for quite some time. Preparation and communication will go a long way in keeping you on track and on time (see "Checklist for Storm Preparation" at the end of this chapter).

Illness or Death

Family Member

Being an online student requires concentration and focused energy to complete assignments and stay on track. Unfortunately, human life does not always cooperate with one's schedule. An illness or death of a family member is undoubtedly one of the most difficult challenges to be faced at any time; however, when there is no wiggle room in your class schedule, these events can cause increased anxiety and frustration. Being faced with this type of challenge during the course of a class necessitates reorganization of priorities. Obviously, the family situation is the main concern, so balancing your class work with family circumstances will take careful and continued planning. Take the time to effectively plan

Death of a Family Member

I chose an online master's program because my aged mother's health was deteriorating and I needed the flexibility of online classes. Two weeks into the start of my program, my mother died. As I was the only sibling living in her town, my brother and sister, along with their families, gathered at my home each day as we did what needed to be done after her death. This required me to provide meals and clean up each day, while still dealing with my overwhelming grief. I considered dropping out of classes, as I was having difficulty keeping up and could not seem to prioritize my work or manage my time. After a couple of days, I knew I had to do some course work or I would never be able to catch up. I sat at the computer, looked at my assignment, and something clicked. I was able to shut out the rest of the world and throw myself mentally into the assignment. It felt so good to do something normal that I realized I needed to keep doing my class work as a respite from my life. It didn't take that long and I felt so much better having accomplished something that was important to me. I also realized my mother would not have wanted me to give up my schooling, so I felt that I was honoring her memory by doing well in the program.

for and address all that needs to be done, keeping in mind that your priorities may be different from those of others. Determine what must be done and what should be done. This will establish your list of priorities and timelines for completion. Accept that you may not be able to do everything on your own, and allow for the delegation of duties that can be sufficiently accomplished by others.

One effective strategy is to write down the five most important things you have to do the next day. List them in order of importance, and when morning comes, begin working on them one by one. Even if you only accomplish one item on your list, it will have been the most important item and the others will have to wait. Look at your list every night before going to sleep and reprioritize as necessary until all of your tasks are completed. This strategy will help to keep your mind focused and assist you in tackling your tasks one by one (Texas Woman's University, 2007b).

Because dealing with the illness or death of a loved one is so stressful and painful, some students may find respite in attending class. Taking time out of your day to put aside the stressor and refocusing your thoughts and energies exclusively on your assignment could provide temporary relief. As you are scheduling your activities for the day, try to set aside at least 30 minutes to concentrate on your class assignment and see if this strategy works for you.

Personal Illness

Serious personal illness is one of the most difficult challenges to face, regardless of whether you are a student or not. When you receive news that you have been diagnosed with a serious illness, a period of disbelief can hinder your planning and thinking abilities. Regardless of your coping abilities and personality, the initial period of discovery must be dealt with and your online program undoubtedly will not be the priority. If the diagnosis is a severe illness that will require prolonged or intense treatment, modification of your study program must be addressed. A discussion with your physician assists in making the adjustments to your studies so that your health and recovery are the primary concerns. It will also be necessary to have a direct discussion with your instructor and advisor at your university. Keep them informed of your treatment plans. Discuss options available in your program that will allow you to both care for yourself and maintain your student responsibilities.

During this difficult time, delegate responsibilities other than your class assignments to anyone and everyone willing to assist you. Your primary responsibility is to yourself and the restoration of your health. Accept help from others for household chores and any family responsibilities you may have, such as child care, running errands, and community functions.

Consider rescheduling your classes. If you find that you are simply too ill to focus on completion of assignments, discuss with your university advisor the possibility of taking a break from your program. Discuss the pros and cons that taking a leave of absence from the program may entail. Learn what is involved in resuming classes when you are feeling capable. This type of preparation will afford you valuable peace of mind during your treatment and a plan for resuming classes upon your recovery.

Traveling During Classes

Remember the days when your instructor would take attendance? That is the beauty of online classes. You can be in attendance no matter where you are in the world. The wrenches in the works, however, are lack of access to a computer and an unreliable Internet connection.

Students choosing an online format for classes claim they embrace the opportunity to take responsibility for their own education as an adult learner and generally find that they are self-disciplined (Thiele, 2003). Traveling during classes, however, may prove to be more of a challenge than anticipated. Travel disrupts your normal daily pattern and can throw your study schedule into chaos. Controlling your learning environment by studying when it is convenient may not work while vacationing or traveling with others. Some may find that scheduling vacations or a trip during previously established semester breaks and university holidays provides the best solution for this challenge. It also can be advantageous to travel midcourse rather than at the beginning or at the end of a class, when you are generally concentrating on getting organized or submitting major projects. Some students may not have the luxury of planning for travel during these times, especially if it is a trip scheduled by others, such as a conference or large group trip. This type of situation is not ideal, but can be dealt with by planning in advance.

If you find travel required during an inopportune time in your class program, consider working a week ahead so that you are free to enjoy your trip without worry about class responsibilities. If this is not an option, research your destination, identifying the availability of Internet access and computers. Many major hotels provide free Internet access or charge a small fee for use, but you may have to carry your own laptop computer as you travel. If you will be aboard a cruise ship or traveling outside the country, your research

Family Vacation

During my 2 years as an online student, I faced challenges with submission of assignments twice due to travel. The first situation was a big family cruise that took us out of the country for a week. Computers were not available on the ship, and, honestly, I was having such a great time that I didn't work on my assignments anyway! I tried to complete my research and work on a major paper prior to the trip, but still had weekly discussions that had to be submitted or I would lose five points. While in port in Mexico, I located an Internet café, rented the computer and Internet time, and completed my discussion assignments. I did not do the best job, but I was at least able to submit something on time.

The other trip was to a remote area in the mountains that did not have Internet access. I had completed my assignments prior to the trip and saved them on a travel drive, but I had to drive to a town that had a library with Internet access so I could submit my assignments. When I arrived at the library, I found that I would need to use their computer to obtain Internet access, so I showed them my driver's license to get a temporary library card and submitted my assignments that day without any further problems.

should identify locations such as Internet cafés or libraries that provide both computers and Internet access. Certain libraries require identification for a temporary library card, but they do not usually charge a fee for computer use. Internet cafés generally charge a reasonable fee for use, based on the time the computer and Internet are utilized.

The most challenging situation is traveling to an area with no Internet access. If you are faced with this situation, your only option is to complete your work early and either submit the work early, if permissible, or have a friend or family member who is not traveling with you upload the assignment when it is due. Whatever arrangements you make for submission based on your advanced planning, do not procrastinate.

Failing a Class

Despite your best planning and effort, the possibility of doing poorly in, or even failing, a class exists. If you find yourself in this situation, it is time for some serious self-reflection on the reason or reasons you have a failing grade. Consider your commitment to the class and your time management strategies. Have you dedicated time at least 3 days a week to your class? If the time or the day you have selected is not working, begin a new strategy immediately. There is no benefit to sticking to a program that is not working.

If time management is not the issue, perhaps it is content in your discussions and papers. Review the class grading rubric including all content necessary to meet the minimum requirements. This necessitates research on your part prior to writing the discussion or paper, but it is time well spent. Start with your topic, conduct your research through peer-reviewed scholarly journals, outline your content, and just start writing. Procrastination swiftly leads you down the road to failure. Think back to when you made the choice to take an online class and remember that most online learners choose this format because they are self-motivated and independent students (O'Neil & Fisher, 2008). If you have lost your motivation and you are unable to rekindle it, perhaps it is time to reach out to fellow students and your instructor. Online instructors realize that their role is vital to the success of the students, and this includes prompt feedback and initiation of communication (Thiele, 2003). The instructor has made the commitment to be there for you and it is your responsibility to utilize that important resource for your success.

Lastly, but certainly not least, fellow students are your best resource. Strive to establish a relationship with your classmates, as they can prove to be a great source of encouragement and information. Many online students have found that help-seeking strategies improve their grades and their enjoyment for online classes, but it is the responsibility of each student to actively engage with other students (Kumrow, 2007). Most online classes offer a student lounge area on the course home page; however, it is the responsibility of the students to initiate communications within that forum. Undoubtedly you will find some students responding regularly, while others are simply not interested. Developing relationships with fellow students leads to socialization, discussions regarding assignments that are unclear, sharing information and references, and encouragement and support when it is most needed. As a result, you may also find that you have developed friendships lasting for many years after the coursework is completed.

Step Up to the Plate

I found that certain students always responded to my classroom discussions and that their thinking was along the same line as mine. They challenged some of my ideas and really made me look in depth at the weekly assignment. Certain responses were so professional and scholarly that I felt the need for improvement in my own work. This realization forced me to step up to the plate and improve both my research and my writing. While the instructor also offered feedback regarding my work, I found my motivation for improvement was the desire to be one of the students writing the excellent discussions that received a large number of responses. Along the way, I discovered that the improved effort in my writing and research led to enhanced learning and better grades. I never would have seen all of the discussion written in my fellow students' papers if I had been in a face-to-face class. What a great learning and motivational tool!

I also noticed that I would log in frequently to the student lounge. I enjoyed becoming friends with my classmates as we discussed school, life, and family. Some of us eventually started communicating outside of the online format and we made plans to meet as a group at graduation. Even now, a year after graduation, we continue to communicate with one another, and I expect this to continue well into the future.

Falling Behind

Despite the best plans, there may be a time when you find you have lost control of your schedule and you are unable to complete your class assignments on time. This situation presents two challenges—catching up and taking steps to prevent it from occurring again. Because most online classes are short, averaging between 6 and 8 weeks with assignments due weekly and projects due before the conclusion of the class, efficient time management is essential.

Let us tackle the first challenge of dealing with falling behind in the submission of weekly assignments. Whatever the reason your study schedule failed, it is better to submit some kind of work rather than none. Although quality is important, it is essential to realize that receiving a zero for the week is not an acceptable solution. When you are close to the end of the week and you have not yet worked on your discussion or posting, it is time to get into high gear and focus on the task at hand. Prioritization is a must. Social and personal events must place second in order to get the work done. Stay calm, sit down at the computer, and concentrate on the assignment. If you are drawing a blank, read the postings of fellow students to stimulate ideas and get involved in the assignment mentally. Take notes as you read the discussions and formulate an idea for your posting. Once you are into the assignment and focusing your thoughts, identify several references supporting your ideas and go to work. Do your best to prevent interruptions until your task is complete and posted. This may require keeping a drink and snack at the computer, unplugging or turning off the phone, or even missing a few hours of sleep. Recruit family members to handle responsibilities until your assignment is complete, reminding them that they too will benefit from these efforts, as you will emerge a happier, calmer person once you hit that last computer key posting your assignment.

Now let us deal with the second part of this challenge: not falling behind again. There is no doubt that adding online courses to your life will require a careful and effective time management program. One method of accomplishing this involves setting modest goals to assist in achieving larger goals. In this case, the larger goal is successfully completing your online class on time. The first step requires planning prior to the start of the class. Most online classes allow access to the syllabus several days prior to the official start date. At that point, look at all your assignments and break them into smaller, manageable units. Estimate the time required to complete each small unit, list the due dates, and set up a weekly schedule. Obviously, the true secret of success is maintaining that weekly schedule. Try limiting extra activities for at least one of the weeks in the class and schedule extra time that week for catch-up, should it be necessary. Other useful suggestions include studying at the same time every day, spacing study periods to maintain productivity, planning for weekly reviews, and leaving some time unscheduled for flexibility (Texas Woman's University, 2007a).

Although stress is common when taking any class or having a deadline for a project, chronic stress can exhaust the body and decrease both the quality and quantity of your work. Poor time management and falling behind in your studies will undoubtedly cause stress for any student. Following the aforementioned suggestions for time management will help to maintain control, reduce stress, and increase productivity (Milliken, Clements, & Tillman, 2007).

Conclusion

The probability of encountering an unexpected challenge while in the online classroom is high. Preparing for the unexpected may be the difference between staying on schedule, falling behind, or perhaps dropping out of class altogether. Before you open your syllabus, take a few moments and consider what may come up during the time you are in class. Whether it is a weather event, a personal crisis, or some other incident, remember to maintain communication with your instructor and classmates. Perform as much as possible during the challenging time and formulate a plan to get back on schedule. Utilize the suggestions contained in this chapter to reduce stress and be prepared. Stay calm, remain organized, and remember that unexpected challenges can be managed with advance preparation and time.

Checklist for Storm Preparation

_______ Arrange for personal and family safety.

_______ Check up on available resources located within community.

_______ Protect computer equipment.

_______ Put printed material in water-tight containers.

_______ Back up assignments on a travel drive.

_______ Get evacuation plan/supplies ready.

_______ Communicate with instructor.

_______ Communicate with classmates.

_______ Complete work ahead of schedule.

_______ Charge laptop battery.

_______ Place all equipment in a crush-proof container.

References

Ferguson, F., Jr., & Watson, D. G. (2003). *Hurricane preparedness and recovery of computer equipment and software.* Retrieved October 20, 2008, from University of Florida Web site: http://edis.ifas.ufl.edu

Kumrow, D. E. (2007). Evidence-based strategies of graduate students to achieve success in a hybrid Web-based course. *Journal of Nursing Education, 46*(3), 140–146.

Milliken, T. F., Clements, P. T., & Tillman, H. J. (2007). The impact of stress management on nurse productivity and retention. *Nursing Economics, 25*(4), 203–211.

O'Neil, C., & Fisher, C. (2008). Should I take this course online? *Journal of Nursing Education, 47*(2), 53–59.

Texas Woman's University. (2007a). *Efficient time scheduling.* Retrieved October 20, 2009, from Counseling Center TWU self-help library Web site: http://www.twu.edu/O-SL/counseling/SelfHelp019.html

Texas Woman's University. (2007b). *Prioritizing.* Retrieved October 20, 2009, from Counseling Center TWU self-help library Web site: http://www.twu.edu/O-sl/counseling/SelfHelp046.html

Thiele, J. E. (2003). Learning patterns of online students. *Journal of Nursing Education, 42*(8), 364–368.

Zsohar, H., & Smith, J. A. (2008). Transition from the classroom to the Web: Successful strategies for teaching online. *Nursing Education Perspectives, 29*(1), 23–29.

Chapter 5

First Class Tips: Beginning Your Online Classroom Experience

Julie Fomenko

In a recent survey of chief academic officers, 62% felt the online learning environment was equal, if not superior, to the classroom environment (Allen & Seaman, 2006). In the book, *The No Significant Difference Phenomenon,* author Thomas Russell compiled 355 research reports noting no differences in the academic achievements of distance learning students as compared to the traditional face-to-face students (Russell, 2001). Regardless of your motivation behind choosing an online format over the traditional environment, all learners must ultimately begin their first day of class.

This chapter provides strategies for online learners to utilize while familiarizing themselves with their first online class. The chapter also offers helpful hints and suggestions from experienced online learners and experienced online faculty. Necessities prior to the beginning of class, such as home, technology, and time requirements, are discussed, and various techniques, both successful and otherwise, are highlighted, providing online students with tools to thrive in the online classroom.

Organizing Yourself for Class

Prior to beginning your class, locate a spot at home that will serve as your classroom desk. This spot should be located in an area where distractions will be kept to an absolute minimum. It should also have adequate light and space. Then, neatly organize your workspace so that essential school items are within easy reach. Keeping things neat and organized can significantly impact your coursework and will make the completion of assignments considerably less stressful. Finally, ensure that you have the required textbooks and associated documents, workbooks, and materials. Depending on the course, other items may also be required to complete your assignments, such as a printer, reference books, computer disks, or other school supplies.

The Computer

Each distance-learning center will provide a list of the technology requirements needed to access the college, the classroom, and the learning resources. To ensure classroom success, you should be proficient in navigating the Internet, in sending and receiving email, and in

> **Learning New Skills!**
>
> During the middle of my degree program, I was required to develop a PowerPoint presentation. I had no prior knowledge of the PowerPoint program and struggled to create an adequate presentation. Late one evening, after several frustrating hours, my 10-year-old son walked by my desk, noted my difficulties, and asked if I needed his help. Not thinking he would be able to offer any assistance, I declined his help, forging ahead. He stood there, watching me wrestle with the program, and finally sat down and took over the laptop. He proceeded to assist me in creating a wonderful presentation, complete with pictures and audio. It was then that I realized my son was part of the techno-generation. I continued to utilize his computer expertise throughout the course of my program.
>
> Do not be afraid to ask for help! The younger generations of students are well versed in technology because they have grown up around computers (Prensky, 2009). They can be a wonderful resource while you learn!

using common desktop software products such as Microsoft Office, Microsoft PowerPoint, Adobe Acrobat Reader, and Windows Media Player. Course-specific requirements will be listed on the class syllabus. If you find that you need more practice with computer literacy and keyboarding, it would be advisable to learn or update these skills prior to entering the online learning environment.

Set Aside a Block of Time

Setting aside a consistent block of time dedicated to coursework provides the regularity necessary for many students to develop the discipline associated with online learning. Many students report spending 10–20 hours a week, per course, on assignments, online discussions, and course reading (eLearners.com, 2008; Walden University, 2008). Following a regular schedule helps students to stay up to date with classroom work.

Getting Started on the Right Foot

By the time you begin your first class, all of the textbooks and required coursework items, such as DVDs, CDs, workbooks, and preprinted articles should be in your possession. If you fail to receive course materials prior to class, contact the institution immediately so as not to delay your coursework. Contact information for frequently asked questions on specific issues, such as missing or incorrect course materials, should be furnished in your admission documents or in your course syllabus.

Organize Course Materials

It is imperative to familiarize yourself with your course as soon as possible. Knowing how to navigate through the class proves invaluable for successful course management. After familiarizing yourself with the course, take the time to organize your course materials. Whether you print out every course document, copy and paste discussion posts into a master document, or just simply read the material, organization can be a make-or-break moment for the class. A good way to handle organization is to place all the material in a three-ring binder and separate the material week by week for easy reference. For example, week 1 would contain the weekly reading assignments, writing assignments, and posting requirements. Week 2, week 3, and so on would contain this information and any other necessary information to successfully complete each week.

Review the Course Syllabus

One of the first items you should familiarize yourself with is the course syllabus. White and Weight (2000) suggest you consider the syllabus as the foundation or framework for your course. This document is designed to inform you of all the class particulars. The syllabus includes a wealth of information such as instructor contact data, course prerequisites, course objectives, course outline, required textbooks and references, course expectations, course policies (including grading criteria), information on how to submit assignments, and links to course resources. The syllabus may also include a course calendar, which may be an entirely separate document. Within the calendar, workload sequencing, reading schedules, project timelines, and assignment due dates should be indicated.

I surveyed over 40 online students and faculty and found the main reason online students experienced difficulties was failure to read the syllabus completely. The best advice I found throughout my coursework and echoed from the survey participants was to read the syllabus.

Get Organized and Stay Organized!

For each class I started, I would immediately print out the course syllabus, course calendar, and grading rubric. I would separate the information and place it into a three-ring binder divided by weeks because each of my courses was 8 weeks long. In this way, I could easily flip to the appropriate week to review coursework, the timeline, and grading rubric to ensure that I completed all the necessary items on time.

Become a Slave to the Calendar!

Whenever I began a new course, I would review the syllabus and all course documents completely. I would then mark on a large calendar that sat by my desk, each and every assignment, project, and paper due date in colored marker. Each assignment had a different color (papers in red, projects/discussion posts in blue, and reading assignments in green). With the timeline in front of me every time I sat down at the computer, I was constantly reminded of the due dates and never failed to turn in an assignment on time.

Get to Know Your Instructor

Most online courses post a biographical sketch of the instructor within the course. It is advisable to become acquainted with your course instructor as you begin class. Many instructors indicate their preferences for how and when students should contact them. This is valuable information that can influence your grade. If your instructor states that he prefers to be emailed, do not call him late at night to pose your question. Make sure you understand how and when to contact your instructor. If you have questions or need clarification after familiarizing yourself with the course syllabus, contact your instructor early on in the program with your concerns in order to ensure you meet the course expectations and objectives.

Access the Student Lounge

Within the electronic classroom, you may find a student lounge. Similar to the student lounge on a traditional college campus, the online lounge is an area within the course designed for students to introduce themselves, ask questions, exchange ideas, and socialize. It is often a place just for students, although the instructor may have access to this area as well.

The student lounge is also a good forum to ask clarifying questions and to get assistance on an assignment from fellow students. It can also be a fun place to hang out with classmates. This type of collaboration can minimize the sense of isolation felt by many online students, while increasing satisfaction with the online experience (Palloff & Pratt, 2003).

Delving Into the Classroom

The Web-based classroom allows students to learn without the typical distractions noted in the traditional classroom such as gum chewing, pencil tapping, or highlights of the night before. This type of classroom also assists those with irregular routines because of shift work as well as those living in time zones other than the one where the school is located. Electronic classrooms can integrate morning and night people, those who must travel, and those with hectic lifestyles that are not conducive to the traditional classroom. Additionally, electronic classrooms tend to increase communication between the students and the instructor (Maeroff, 2003).

Homework and Pj's!

One of my favorite things about the online classroom was the ability to attend class in my pajamas. Working full-time as a night shift nurse, I was often up at 3 or 4 a.m. posting, making comments to other students, or proofreading my papers. I did not have to worry about the typical classroom distractions and could simply concentrate on my studies. Having the flexibility of time, I was able to complete much of my coursework while my family slept, and this flexibility of the online classroom environment allowed me to complete my master's degree. With my family and work requirements, I doubt I would have been able to complete a master's program in the traditional classroom setting.

Discussion Board

The discussion board is a huge component of many online classes. Timed discussion posts are assigned by the instructor, typically each week, with a particular topic or question posed to the class. You may be asked to support or oppose a controversial topic, highlight current research on a subject, summarize a theory, or simply discuss your personal opinion. The discussion post requirements should be clearly defined within the syllabus or course assignment. The class may have a requisite number of posts each week, or a requisite number of replies to other students' posts. Be sure to know exactly what your weekly posting requirements entail.

Submitting Assignments

When the time comes to turn assignments in to the instructor, it is imperative that you understand the how and when of submitting them. Many classrooms have a virtual drop box. This is an electronic mailbox where students submit assignments. The drop box should time stamp and date stamp your assignments, so be aware of the due dates. Alternatively, some instructors may want assignments emailed to them. Make sure you understand how to transmit documents electronically. Students should become comfortable with their ability to mail attachments, upload document files, create PDF documents, and construct spreadsheets in order to get the deliverables turned in on time. You do not want your hard work ending up missing somewhere in cyberspace.

Group Projects

In the traditional classroom, group projects are common and easy to arrange. The group members select a time and place to meet and work together to complete the project. Group projects are also a part of many online courses, but the group must come together in a different manner. Chat rooms and blackboards are common in today's virtual classroom. Comparable to the traditional setting, groups choose a date and time to meet. This meeting is similar to a conference call. Each group member logs in to the chat room at the selected time and members can talk to each other via instant messaging. You may even have access to the virtual blackboard where members can draw and diagram elements of the project. Virtual blackboards are a useful and fun tool when utilized appropriately, and can help to ensure each member of the team completes his or her assigned work component.

> **Blackboards and Hangman**
>
> During one of my group projects, our group frequently met to complete our assignment in the chat room. In the chat room, we could brainstorm and integrate everyone's ideas. It was a great way to have real-time conversations and discuss our work. However, the real fun started when we tried out the blackboard. The blackboard was an electronic chalkboard to write and draw on, using the computer mouse. Two of us started to draw out our ideas, which soon digressed into a game of hangman. We managed to complete the project, and my drawing partner and I remain good friends to this day.

Alternate E-Classroom Communication

Your classroom may utilize other options for communications, such as streaming video, teleconferencing, and conference calls. As a student, you can remain at home where you feel comfortable and safe, while still participating with people from all over the world. Be sure to understand which forms of communications are offered and required for your class. This information should be noted in the class syllabus or through communications with your instructor.

Friendships

The most gratifying piece of my virtual classroom experience involved the close friendships I made with a group of wonderful women. It was amazing to me how much we all bonded during our 2-year program. We discussed coursework, argued points of contention, debated the pros and cons of a subject, commiserated when times were tough, and celebrated victories. We "met" for coffee online, proofread each other's assignments, and simply supported one another. These women remain close friends of mine to this day. Not only did I receive my master's degree, but I was also blessed with amazing friends through my online course of study.

Grade Book

The grade book is the section of your classroom where your instructor posts your grades and class scores. The grade book is commonly used by the instructor to post scores for submitted assignments. Typically, individual grades are kept confidential and are posted only for individual student viewing. However, instructors may post the range of class scores for a specific assignment without specifying student identity. Certain instructors may send scores to personal email accounts as well. Familiarize yourself with the grading policy for your specific instructor and institution.

Bear in mind that not all institutions or instructors follow similar grading rubrics. In many instances, an 83 is no longer a "B," but a "C." Frequently, graduate programs require a minimum grade in order to fulfill course requirements. Understand and familiarize yourself with your institutions grading rubric to avoid potential confusion and disappointment.

Conclusion

Beginning an online class or program offers many advantages to you as a student. You have the freedom to learn wherever and whenever you choose. You can stay in your pajamas sipping coffee or stay up late after your children are in bed in order to complete your assignments. You can take your classroom along on vacation or business travel and work when you have the opportunity. You can network with other like-minded people and discover new friendships, while earning the degree you have always wanted and completing it on your timetable. Your options are as endless as your imagination. If you are ready to advance your personal education, work towards a professional promotion, or get your degree, the virtual classroom may be just the option for which you've been waiting. Good luck in your studies!

FIGURE 5-1 Tips for Beginning Online Students

Do . . .

- Research the institution and coursework.
- Become familiar with required technology and tools.
- Read the syllabus thoroughly.
- Dedicate work space for coursework.
- Know due dates.
- Ask questions when uncertain.
- Use available assistance (writing centers, counselors, etc.).
- Dedicate a specific time for coursework.
- Collaborate with like-minded students.

Do not . . .

- Fail to read required course documents.
- Fail to keep up with coursework.
- Miss deadlines.
- Be disorganized.
- Fail to take coursework seriously.

Checklist for Beginning Your First Class

______ Locate a spot at home that will serve as your classroom desk.

______ Neatly organize your desk space.

______ Establish a consistent block of time for coursework.

______ Check that you received the appropriate textbooks and course materials.

______ Familiarize yourself with the course as soon as possible.

______ Organize your course materials.

______ Review the course syllabus.

______ Get to know your instructor.

______ Access the student lounge.

______ Take a classroom tour:

- ______ Find the discussion board or chat room.
- ______ Understand how, when, and where to submit assignments.
- ______ Understand how to manage group projects, if required in your course of study.
- ______ Understand what other forms of communication you will be using:
  - ______ Streaming video
  - ______ Teleconference
  - ______ Conference calls

______ Familiarize yourself with the grading policy and grading rubric.

References

Allen, I. E., & Seaman, J. (2006). *Making the grade: Online education in the United States* (pp. 15–16). Needham, MA: Sloan Consortium.

eLearners.com. (2008). *You are ready to go back to school if* . . . Retrieved January 24, 2009, from http://www.elearners.com/guide-to-online-education/you-are-ready-to-go-back-to-school.asp?nl=6

Maeroff, G. I. (2003). *A classroom of one: How online learning is changing our schools and colleges.* New York: Palgrave MacMillan.

Palloff, R. M., & Pratt, K. (2003). *The virtual student: A profile and guide to working with online learners.* San Francisco: Jossey-Bass.

Prensky, M. (2009). *Young minds, fast times: The twenty-first-century digital learner.* Retrieved January 23, 2009, from http://www.edutopia.org/ikid-digital-learner-technology-2008

Russell, T. L. (2001). *The no significant difference phenomenon* (5th ed.). Littleton, CO: International Distance Learning Certification Center.

Walden University. (2008). *About online learning.* Retrieved January 23, 2009, from http://www.walden.edu/c/About/About_237.htm

White, K. W., & Weight, B. H. (2000). *The online teaching guide: A handbook of attitudes, strategies, and techniques for the virtual classroom.* Needham Heights, MA: Allyn & Bacon.

Chapter 6

Tips and Strategies for Successful Writing in the Online Classroom

Michelle Feavel

The ability to communicate ideas and viewpoints effectively in the online learning environment can prove quite challenging for the online student. It is not unusual for students taking online courses to spend a great percentage of their study time developing academic essays and postings (Booth, 1996; Clay, 2003). Lacking the ability to approach the instructor in a face-to-face fashion, the online student is confronted with the fundamental task of clear and concise communication. Indeed, many college students, especially those in the online environment, find the task of writing assignments intimidating, having either a lack of confidence or experience in their writing skills. Nevertheless, with careful preparation and dedication, the online student can successfully overcome these barriers and learn to write effective and concise essays, postings, and responses essential to the online classroom learning experience.

In this chapter, you will become acquainted with the processes and resources involved in developing successful writing habits. Organizing your workspace, accessing the abundant resources available for reference, understanding the variety of computer programs and online resources available to assist you, gaining insight into essential guidelines for writing effective online communications, and the process of approaching a writing assignment are discussed. Your ability to communicate your thoughts effectively, concisely, cohesively, and in a scholarly fashion has a direct influence on your capacity to succeed in the online learning environment. Remember, just as there are numerous approaches to developing writing skills, it is important that each and every student develop his or her own personal writing style, understanding as well that individual instructors will have specific requirements and guidelines influencing these styles. Keeping these ideas in mind will add to your writing success in the online classroom environment.

Getting Started

Organization

It is no secret that organization of a work area will lead to greater productivity. Students, whether in the traditional or online environment, require dedicated space in order to effectively approach assignments. It is essential that you find a place in your home specifically for your online studies, strategically situated away from everyday distractions. Obviously your computer, printer, and textbooks will comprise the focal area of your study space. Have essential materials such as sticky notes, highlighting pens, note cards, spare ink cartridges, printer paper, and file folders readily available. Keep the area free of extraneous clutter, such as mail, newspapers, and household projects. You will find that scholarly writing requires absolute focus on the task at hand, so keep distractions to a minimum. Set up your area in order to keep the flow of ideas and information suited to your writing style. Reference materials should be kept at your fingertips. Purchase portable thumb drives or compact discs for your computer to store and back up valuable data and assignments. Organizing your study area to your specific needs and desires requires an initial time investment; on the other hand, your efforts will be rewarded with increased efficiency and productivity.

Along with organizing your study space, develop a schedule dedicated to your writing efforts. Assign a specified time each day, even if only for 1 hour, to work on your assignments. Students may find it helpful to break down difficult or lengthy writing assignments into more manageable fragments, such as composing a page or a topic per day until the assignment is complete. Take the time to enter assignment deadlines on a calendar that is within full view of your work area. Constant reinforcement of assignment deadlines helps students to develop strategic timetables and avoid last-minute panic. Once you acquire the habit of mapping assignments on a calendar, devising manageable schedules and timetables will become second nature. The practice of working toward manageable goals assists with handling the stress that comes with deadlines.

Creative Organization

My daughter developed a very interesting method of keeping an assignment calendar. She lived in an apartment that had a very large, mirrored wall next to her study area. She purchased a variety of different colored grease pencils and would write her assignment calendar on the mirrored wall with these pencils. Different courses were color-coded, allowing her to discern at a glance which assignments were due on specific dates. Assignments could be easily updated by cleaning the mirror! Obviously, a white board will work just as effectively if you do not have a mirrored wall!

Reference Sources

Taking the time to think about and examine what is required in a writing assignment is fundamental to producing a successful essay (Booth, 1996). It is essential for you to understand exactly what your instructor expects from the writing experience. Essay assignments require critical thinking, assessment, analysis, and support of ideas in an intellectual and unbiased fashion. In order to accomplish these goals, you need the information and support available in current literature references.

Once you are clear on the subject or topic of your essay, the hunt for relevant literature can begin. This is not as simple as it may sound. There are literally thousands of professional journals, scholarly articles, textbooks, and CDs available for reference. Choosing the appropriate support literature can make a world of difference in the quality of your essay. The following tips will help guide you to determine what each has to offer.

Tip No. 1: Textbooks

Obviously a list of textbooks will be provided by your course instructor. Textbooks can be an excellent reference source, provided they have been published within a recent time frame. Remember, information on a variety of topics, particularly those in healthcare policy and information technology fields, is constantly being updated. It is advisable to utilize your textbooks as basic references. However, many instructors like to see their students expand beyond the textbook realm and move into periodical literature to support their writing. This demonstrates the ability on your part to think critically and apply your knowledge effectively to the issues or subjects involved. Few instructors want their students to regurgitate material presented in textbooks. Your textbooks should serve as a foundation for your writing, providing you with a framework for your assignments. Utilize textbook references sparingly and appropriately, and expand on your knowledge gained from textbooks with information from professional journals, periodicals, and reliable Web sites.

Tip No. 2: Internet and Online Databases

Online students are strongly encouraged to develop familiarity with online search engines and databases in order to broaden their learning base. Engaging in a computerized search related to your assignment topic is a good way to collect valid information to support your subject. Be careful, however, when choosing your information source. Databases such as CINAHL, OVID, ProQuest, MedLine, and those provided by your online institution carry professional and scholastic journals offering an abundance of valid, relevant articles and research for your assignments. Beware of information gained from sites that serve as forums for individuals to post their opinions or invalidated studies. Make sure all of the information you utilize in your writing can be substantiated and is taken from reputable sources. You must be selective when deciding which literature to include in your research. Ask yourself questions, such as:

- Can this author be regarded as authoritative and unbiased?
- Does this author clearly articulate his perspective and provide evidence to support his perspective?
- Do the author's findings contribute knowledge to the subject?
- Does the author address the important issues and questions related to the topic? (Booth, 1996)

Students with limited scholarly writing and research experience may be drawn to utilize the online, free encyclopedia, Wikipedia. Most universities, however, strongly discourage students from utilizing Wikipedia as a valid reference source. In fact, there are certain universities that have specifically banned their students from utilizing Wikipedia citations (Wikipedia, n.d.). Critics of Wikipedia charge that many Wikipedia authors do not have degrees or valid credentials recognized in the world of academia, thus creating an accuracy and reliability issue. Additionally, there are those who feel the information presented in Wikipedia is biased, inconsistent, and easily subject to the addition of unverified information (Wikipedia). Remember, information presented in Wikipedia can be edited by anyone who enters the Web site. Generally speaking, this is not the type of information that lends itself to scholarly writing. Be selective about which reference material you decide to include in your writing assignment. Make sure that your assignment demonstrates independent thought supported by solid evidence rather than merely a collection of borrowed ideas (Booth, 1996). Download articles from the database and highlight specific references you feel are useful to your assignment. Keep in mind it is easy to get bogged down with the voluminous number of reference materials available. You can find yourself drowning in a sea of research if you do not carefully and selectively limit yourself to the number of references you will use. Writing succinct and scholarly papers and postings is key to academic achievement.

Tip No. 3: Professional Journals

Scholastic journals provide a wealth of information for students. It is important that you distinguish scholastic and professional journals from professional magazines. Journals contain timely research information while magazines typically contain editorials and articles unsupported by evidence. Journals are peer reviewed; that is, the research articles contained in them have been reviewed and given validation by other professionals in the author's stated field of study. The information presented in scholastic and professional journals is considered reliable and relevant to their profession and worthy of consideration and support for professional practice. You will find that journals provide not only examination of an issue, but also a wide variety of perspectives on that issue. It is important to compare and contrast various authors' perspectives on a topic, as this demonstrates your ability to think critically and apply the knowledge gained from the journal article. Stay away from editorials and opinion pieces. While the author may be able to support his or her view, opinion/editorial pieces represent bias in thinking. In general, magazine articles hold little influence in scholarly writing. Stick with professional journals.

Tip No. 4: Community/School Libraries

If your online college does not have access to professional databases, you may want to try your public library. Numerous libraries have access to professional databases and offer these services free of charge to their members. Some libraries allow members to access these databases from their homes, while others require on-site usage. Additionally, most public libraries subscribe to a large volume of professional journals. Be sure to enlist the advice and assistance of the librarian in order to direct your search as efficiently as possible.

Tip No. 5: Writing Centers

Your online college may offer writing assistance for its students in the form of a writing center. These centers offer advice, assistance, and tutoring for students having difficulty writing scholarly papers. If you find yourself consistently struggling to compose a scholarly paper, you may want to consider taking a basic writing course. Your online college may offer a freshman-level writing course or a basic writing refresher course reviewing fundamentals for students reentering the collegiate environment. These courses can prove extremely helpful for students who are fraught with anxiety over writing assignments.

Computer Literacy

Now that you have decided to engage in online learning, it is essential that you possess a fundamental working knowledge of computer word processing. Your ability to function in a variety of word processing formats has a direct influence on your success in the online collegiate environment. All word processing programs evolve around basic concepts that must be understood in order to utilize the programs efficiently and effectively. Microsoft Word is probably the most common word processing program utilized in the online collegiate environment; however, other word processing programs are available. Microsoft PowerPoint, while not a word processing program, is worth familiarizing yourself with as many online programs require students to create presentations as a part of their coursework.

Microsoft Word

Word allows you to format your paper, create, save, and edit a document, check for spelling errors, check grammar, and check punctuation. Microsoft Word will enable you to submit written assignments formatted to your instructor's specific requirements easily and effortlessly *if* you understand how the program works! If you are not adept with this word processing program, you will undoubtedly experience a high degree of frustration in attempting your writing assignments. Those individuals who have limited experience using word processing programs should consider updating their skills prior to enrolling in online classes. Many local junior colleges offer short courses in word processing competency. You can also purchase instructional materials if you prefer the do-it-yourself path. Whatever you decide, make it a point to become competent in the word processing program of your choice prior to starting your online courses. You will be glad you did!

Learn to Type!

The greatest limitation of any word processing program is the speed at which you enter the data. This means that the ability to type quickly is extremely valuable. There are many computer-based programs available to assist you in learning how to type. Practicing for as little as a half an hour daily can sharpen your keyboarding skills in as little as 2 weeks. This investment of your time will more than pay for itself in the long run (Grauer & Barber, 1997).

Microsoft PowerPoint

PowerPoint enables the user to develop a professional presentation on the computer. Given the fact that many college instructors utilize presentation development in their courses to prepare students for the business world, it is wise to acquaint yourself with PowerPoint and its many functions. With PowerPoint, you can format your presentation in a variety of creative ways, developing exciting and innovative methods to present your ideas and information. Fortunately, PowerPoint is very easy to learn because you can apply much of what you know from Word to this program. Instructional materials are easily available for PowerPoint as well.

Data Management

Many students will enroll in more than one course per term in their online education experience. Keeping your coursework and information in an orderly fashion, while continuously maintaining easy access to this information, can be challenging. Organizing and maintaining data files for each class will keep necessary information right at your fingertips as well as provide easy future reference.

It is easy to file your work on your computer hard drive. However, as many students have discovered, an unfortunately timed electrical storm or a spilled cup of coffee on a computer keyboard can be a costly event, not only in dollars and cents but in the loss of hard work. Purchase one or two thumb drives or a stack of blank compact discs and back up all of your scholastic computer files. Organize each class separately, according to the class number and term. Within each class, organize your assignments by weeks or by assignment names in order to retrieve information easily. Many thumb drives come color-coded; use a different color for each term. If you use a compact disc to back up your work, you can write your class information directly on the disc. It is important to keep your filing system consistent. Do not change your methodology for filing several different times. Stick to one specific method and apply this method without fail. Always back up your work on the thumb drive or the compact disc at the end of each day. There is no heartache quite like the one caused by lost or irretrievable hard work! Unfortunately, this is one lesson frequently learned the hard way by online students.

Format Aids

It is not difficult to imagine the potential chaos created by thousands of students submitting scholarly works to their instructors without a consistent format. Clear, concise communication, in any venue, requires formatting standards. Formatting provides uniformity in the writing process and allows for efficiency and clear understanding of the written word (American Psychological Association, 2001). The majority of college students are required to submit their writing assignments in some manner or variety of formalized format, such as APA, MLA, or AMA. These formats are based on set rules and requirements formulated to ensure the standardization of written documents and simplify the task of the reader.

For many students, mastering the art of formatting written assignments does not come easily. Format styles are accompanied by format manuals, typically several hundred pages thick! In this age where communication texting has become an art form, it is no surprise that students experience frustration in the application of rigid formatting to their writing assignments.

There exist several ways to approach this issue. The first, and most basic, is to become familiar with the formatting manual. The manual acts as an excellent reference source; however, for students who have minimal exposure to scholarly writing, learning how to format a paper by reading the manual can take longer than writing the assignment itself. Instruction manuals are the ultimate authority for correctly formatting written assignments. Many students, though, find it difficult to retain all of the information contained in the instruction manual. It is useful to find the most frequently used applications, such as margin requirements, heading requirements, table preparation, figure checklists, and a sample paper, and mark these sections with sticky tabs. When you have given this aspect of writing time and practice, formatting your written work will come as second nature.

Students may also find that working through a formatting manual is cumbersome and time consuming. Pressing deadlines for assignment submissions along with searching through bulky formatting manuals can make even the most patient student fraught with anxiety. Fortunately, many colleges and university have online formatting sites that are readily available and provide formatting information in an easy-to-understand design. These sites address frequently asked questions (FAQs), provide examples for virtually any formatting question, and are easy to navigate. For example, Purdue University provides the OWL Resource APA Formatting and Style Guide online at http://owl.english.purdue.edu/owl/resource/560/10/ (Neyhart, Karper, Seas, & Russell, 2008). This Web site is open to anyone wishing to obtain APA formatting information or clarification. I cite this example simply because I have utilized it as a reference. There are, however, numerous colleges and universities that offer similar Web sites that are open for any user. Spend the time visiting various formatting Web sites and find one that you feel is easy to use, addresses your needs, and provides up-to-date information. Make sure that the Web site has been updated recently, as changes in formatting and media reference material occur frequently.

Another method available to ease formatting issues for students is computer software. Rather than become entangled in the formatting web, many students choose to purchase software that automatically formats their papers as they type. Formatting aids can accomplish such tasks as automatically formatting the reference list, creating headers and page numbers, setting up proper margins and line spacing, creating title and abstract pages, formatting headings, providing table templates in which the author simply inserts his or her data, and the list goes on! Students frustrated by formatting issues have turned to software in order to produce the desired outcomes for their assignments. For the most part, these software programs provide accurate templates and minimize the confusion that so often accompanies formatting.

APA the Easy Way!

My undergraduate program in nursing required that all papers be submitted in APA format. Never having utilized any type of formatting before, I found myself drowning in the rules and requirements of APA. My first written assignment was returned to me completely dissected due to APA errors! Although my instructors had warned against utilizing purchased APA software, I decided to take a chance and purchased a program. While this program did not catch every APA error, it significantly improved the quality of my formatting. What the program did not catch I easily corrected myself, and from that point forward I never had a paper returned due to formatting errors. It was money well spent!

However, you must be cautious regarding the software you choose. Be aware that many free templates or guidelines can be acquired on the Internet. This bargain software may be worth exactly what you pay for it. Read reviews for the software you are considering acquiring. Ask friends and colleagues if they have utilized formatting software. Most software programs are available for purchase in the $20–$50 range. The cost varies with the complexity of the software. Be sure to check with your instructors if they have any issues with utilizing formatting software. Certain instructors, especially in the online learning environment, request students refrain from utilizing this software, as it may be incompatible with their computer grading software.

Generally speaking, formatting software has helped many students overcome their angst and frustration with writing scholarly papers. It also allows students to focus more on the content of their assignments than on the format.

Composing the Scholarly Posting/Essay

Writing an academic paper is often a source of apprehension and frustration for college students. Evidence suggests that writing remains a source of concern for many college students as they lack the understanding of how to approach the writing process (Booth, 1996; Clay, 2003). The online environment can magnify the problem due simply to the fact that the student/instructor relationship is based more on an independent level rather than on a supervisory level. Students are encouraged to branch out on their own, seeking information with a minimal amount of oversight from the instructor. Given the fact that online students will spend an excessive amount of time composing postings and essays for their courses, it is of vital importance to understand and utilize the writing process. Developing a strategic approach to academic writing assignments will ensure the effectiveness and accuracy of the assignment, as well as bolstering students' confidence in approaching the assignment (Clay).

Planning

You may find yourself eager to plunge directly into a writing assignment, simply concerned with finishing the project rather than approaching it in a logical, systematic fashion. Spending time thinking carefully about your topic and examining your approach is exactly what is required for producing a quality essay (Booth, 1996; Clay, 2003; Lee, 2003). Academic writing requires a critical approach and should not simply be a summary of relevant literature (Booth). Once you have a clear image of the assignment, a collection of relevant literature is the next step. Booth recommends carrying out a computer search as a good way to begin. Formulate a set of questions regarding your essay or posting before you start. Ask yourself questions, such as what you need to reveal about your topic in your writing, what assertions you must support, what type of parallels you must draw, and how many, if any, varying perspectives you should include. Including an analysis of this sort will demonstrate a level of critical thinking in your writing. Steer away from biased, unsupported opinions, unless of course the basis of your essay is editorial in nature. Strong, unbiased, and peer-reviewed research facts should form the basis of your essay.

Booth (1996) suggests that at this stage, all information necessary to your essay be available. Highlight areas of your references you wish to include in your writing. If your writing style requires a more disciplined approach, write note cards with the essay information and author information and file them in the order to be addressed in your essay. Place a time limit on yourself for gathering your research information; otherwise you may become bogged down in the mire of collecting material and deciding which information is relevant to your essay.

Organizing Your Ideas

The next step is to organize the ideas for your essay into an outline. The purpose behind the outline is to create a structured and logical approach to your topic and provide you with a map to stay on target. Your outline should be divided into the following three basic parts: the introduction, the main body, and the conclusion.

Introduction

The introduction tells the reader what will be presented in the essay. Depending on the length of your essay, your introduction should mention each of the issues you intend to identify in the main body of your essay and comprise one to two paragraphs. The issues should be listed as they are presented in your essay. As suggested by Booth, your introduction may include:

- A question that will be answered later
- A statement of the case to be argued
- An outline of the reasons for focusing on specific aspects of a general topic
- A selection of data to establish that an issue is worth discussing
- A quotation that conveys the key ideas to be discussed

It is fundamental that your introduction provide the reader with the main focus of your essay. An overview of the issues you will discuss and the reasons why, and a summary of how the essay will develop the topic gives the reader essential guidance in understanding your essay (Booth, 1996). A good concept for formatting your introduction is to link the conclusion to the main findings. For example, the following statement could be incorporated into an introduction:

> This paper will provide a practical overview on the process of writing a scholarly essay. Elements essential to organization, planning, and composing the essay will be described.

It is not necessary to compose your essay in the exact order of the outline. Composition is not a linear process, where you start at the introduction and end with the conclusion (Clay, 2003). Often times the introduction is best written after you have completed your essay. Many students experience writer's block when attempting to compose a paper in a linear fashion. Write about the issues identified in your essay as you think about them, and then put them in the order you have identified. As long as the final product adheres to the developed outline, you may be surprised at how easily your essay takes form (Clay).

Main Body

The main body is where your central ideas and arguments take shape. This is the crux of your essay. This portion should guide the reader, taking him easily from one section to the next; therefore, the main body should develop logically and analytically (Booth, 1996). Each paragraph should be based on the issues you have identified in your outline and introduction and contain references from your literature search. Remember to limit the content of the paragraph to one main topic, with the first line of your paragraphs introducing the topic to be discussed. Where two paragraphs address different aspects of the same topic, link the two together with phrases such as "in addition to . . ." or "in a similar fashion . . ." (Clay, 2003). Avoid using terminology you do not understand or are unfamiliar with. This only serves to confuse the reader. Use short, comprehensible sentences that are easily understood (Clay). Make sure the essay flows in a logical sequence and leads clearly to the conclusion (Booth, 1996). Stay focused on your outline to avoid wandering off topic.

Conclusion

The conclusion represents the summary of the ideas presented in your paper; in other words, you should tell the reader what you just told them. The conclusion should never introduce new material. In order to demonstrate critical thinking, provide an analysis of the issues rather than simply restating facts already presented in the essay. Conclusions should be written in the past tense, using phrases such as "this paper has demonstrated that . . ." and "evidence clearly suggests that . . ." (Clay, 2003). Consider including such implications as future trends or ideas for consideration (Booth, 1996). If, upon review of your essay, you notice material in your conclusion that was not approached in the body of your essay, simply cut these items from the conclusion and paste them in the body of the essay as new paragraphs. You may also find that these topics are not relevant to the crux of the essay, in which case you can discard them or simply file these topics away for future reference (Booth). Limit your conclusion to one or two paragraphs. The need for a conclusion of greater length indicates you have not developed your topic fully in the body of the essay.

> **Happy Endings!**
>
> Here's a tip for writing the conclusion to your essay. Booth (1996) suggests using a highlighter to mark the most important point of each paragraph in your essay. Then link each of these findings together to develop your conclusion.

Revisions

Many students find it difficult, if not impossible, to compose an essay to their satisfaction on the first attempt. In fact, it is suggested that once you complete the first draft of your essay, you should step back and review your work. Pace your essay construction to allow yourself time for review and editing. Producing an early first draft of your essay allows for a few days to set the paper aside in order to gain fresh perspective when proofreading. You may find, however, that you have become so engrossed in your own work that engaging in an unbiased critique is difficult at best. If this is the case, seek critical feedback from a friend or classmate to provide helpful insight. Perhaps your instructor would be open to previewing your essay and providing supportive tips on how it could be improved. Bear in mind that it is easy for you to follow the logic of your essay because you wrote and developed it. Obtaining the critical perspective of another will help establish where your essay meets its objectives or demonstrates weakness.

When proofreading, ask yourself the following questions:

- Does my essay satisfy the assignment criteria and guidelines?
- Are there run-on sentences or sentences that lack subject/verb agreement?
- Are there words that are overused? Use your thesaurus to substitute similar words for those that are used too frequently.
- Are my references relevant and current?
- Are my references cited correctly?
- Is my essay unbiased?
- Are there mistakes in punctuation?
- Does my essay flow smoothly from one paragraph to the next?

Proofread your essay aloud. This enables you to decide if the punctuation is correct and determine whether or not the material flows consistently and congruently (Clay, 2003). Bear in mind that virtually all written material, even that composed by professionals, must endure editing and numerous revisions. Be sure to file for future reference all suggestions, corrections, and helpful hints provided by your instructor. Keep a copy of your graded or critiqued essays. These essays are figuratively worth their weight in gold when composing future assignments!

Support

The online learning environment fosters and encourages independence in students. However, many students in the beginning of their online experience may feel the need for the support, camaraderie, and guidance typically found in the traditional classroom. This is particularly true when it comes to writing assignments. The importance of the student/instructor relationship cannot be emphasized more emphatically than in the online environment. Seek out faculty assistance and clarification for assignments. Ask the instructor for contact information if it is not provided. Do not hesitate to contact your instructor when you feel instructions are ambiguous or confusing. Be specific when asking questions. Consider posting questions relevant to the entire class on classroom bulletin boards or mailboxes. Make certain that all instructions for the assignment are answered to your satisfaction. Your comfort and success in the online classroom depend upon your commitment to open communication.

Don't neglect to tap into a readily available resource—your fellow classmates. You may find that working in groups provides a level of support and assurance that you need. Perhaps certain members of your online classroom have been in this environment before or have workplace experience relevant to your course of study. Certain students may have a flair for critiquing writing or have the ability to assist others when they feel they have run into a brick wall. Others may have access to different online libraries or additional reference sites. Develop relationships with your classmates, if not for the academic support, then for the emotional support. Online classrooms can be as interactive as traditional classrooms. It is up to you to make it the experience you desire.

Classroom Dynamics

During my online graduate course experience I was fortunate to develop friendships with a specific group of fellow nurses. We formed a bond that exists to this day! We offered each other support during finals and otherwise difficult courses, shared our learning experiences, provided each other with advice on specific instructors, and generally helped each other get through trying times of juggling family, work, and school assignments. We would read each other's papers and offer suggestions. Those who were computer aficionados helped those who were not. We would find reference material in our hospital libraries and share with those who did not have libraries at their workplace. In short, these friendships proved invaluable, both in and out of the classroom, and helped each of us succeed in our chosen academic goals.

Conclusion

Developing and mastering the ability to write academic essays and postings is essential to your classroom achievement. While challenging, the art of writing a scholarly essay or posting can be acquired if approached in a logical and patient fashion. The confidence demonstrated in your writing ability will undoubtedly improve with each assignment. The tools, skills, and tips presented in this chapter will assist you in successfully managing the writing process. Realize that the art of written communication is your main conduit to success in the online environment. Practice, discipline, attention to detail, and perseverance will pay off in well-written essays and postings worthy of the online collegiate student!

Checklist for Composing a Successful Essay

_______ Develop a timetable. Make specific goals and assign specific dates for the completion of these goals.

_______ Define the topic. Understand/verify the specific topic or subject of the essay.

_______ Formulate a set of questions regarding the topic. Decide how you want to approach the topic.

_______ Perform the research for your topic. Obtain scholarly, relevant research material to support your questions.

_______ Develop an outline (introduction/body/conclusion). Highlight areas of reference material to be included in your essay and organize this information in accordance with your outline.

_______ Produce a rough draft.

_______ Review/revise your rough draft. Ask yourself the following questions regarding your draft:

- _______ Does my essay satisfy the assignment criteria and guidelines?
- _______ Are there run-on sentences or sentences that lack subject/verb agreement?
- _______ Are there words that are overused? Use your thesaurus to substitute similar words for those that are used too frequently.
- _______ Are my references relevant and current?
- _______ Are my references cited correctly?
- _______ Is my essay unbiased?
- _______ Are there mistakes in punctuation?
- _______ Does my essay flow smoothly from one paragraph to the next?

_______ Produce a final copy.

References

American Psychological Association. (2001). *Publication manual of the American Psychological Association* (5th ed.). Washington, DC: Author.

Booth, Y. (1996). Writing an academic essay: A practical guide for nurses. *British Journal of Nursing, 5*(16), 12–25.

Clay, G. (2003). Assignment writing skills. *Nursing Standard, 17*(20), 47–52. Retrieved November 29, 2008 from MedLine database.

Grauer, R. T., & Barber, M. (1997). *Exploring Microsoft Office 97 Professional.* Upper Saddle River, NJ: Prentice Hall.

Lee, P. (2003). Writing academically: Using existing knowledge to improve writing style. *Pediatric Nursing, 15*(7), 47–49. Retrieved December 8, 2008, from EBSCO database.

Neyhart, D., Karper, E., Seas, K., & Russell, T. (2008). *OWL resource. APA formatting and style guide.* Retrieved December 8, 2008, from http://owl.english.purdue.edu/owl/resource/560/10

Wikipedia. (n.d.). *Criticism of Wikipedia.* Retrieved December 6, 2008, from http://en.wikipedia.org/wiki/Criticism_of_Wikipedia

Chapter 7

Formatting: APA, MLA, AMA . . .

Sally Rudy

William Goldman said, "The easiest thing to do on earth is not write" (Nordquist, 2009, para. 7). When asked about the most frightening thing he had ever encountered, novelist Ernest Hemingway said, "A blank sheet of paper" (Nordquist, 2009, para. 5). Summoning the motivation to begin the writing process can be, at best, a struggle. Whether you are stuck on content or proper formatting, the first few words are often the hardest. Although the content of the paper is up to you, the appearance of your work is frequently more than half the battle of writing. This chapter will present information and offer advice that will help you tackle those papers and complete them with proper formatting. The formatting information in this chapter will enable you to create beautiful papers every time you sit down to write, whether for school or for submission to a prestigious peer-reviewed journal. You will have a consistent plan and helpful tools that you can use to facilitate your writing.

Getting Started

In order to thwart writer's block, you should establish a method of writing that is easy, organized, and consistent. Start with an outline or the rubric from your class syllabus, and complete the title page of your work. Then, add the headings from your outline or rubric, including the reference page. The headings do not need to be creative; they can be simply an idea of what you want to write about in that section. In fact, they can even be the same words found in your outline or rubric, which may allow your instructor or editor to easily recognize and identify key topics. Using the rubric headings can improve your grade by demonstrating that you did indeed meet the requirements for the paper by addressing all topics. As you write this skeleton paper, utilize the basic guidelines for formatting a paper in whatever style is required by your college or university or the journal to which you are submitting work.

Having this simple framework down on paper can provide the motivation for you to complete the project (see Figure 7-1). This start also allows you to recognize that you can, in fact, write this paper or article. This realization can preclude that all-too familiar feeling of incapacity—you know, the one that is often accompanied by tears of frustration. With the foundation of the project laid out on paper, you can then apply information from the articles, books, and online information that you have already researched to add the content of your paper. By adding your citations to the reference page as you write, your paper can be

FIGURE 7-1 Skeleton Template for Papers

Running Head:
EXAMPLE 1

Example Skeleton Paper
Sally Rudy, MSN, RN
Penn State Hershey Medical Center
Department of Nursing Education
February 2, 2009

EXAMPLE 2

Abstract

This skeleton template is formatted using the 6th edition of the *Publication Manual of the American Psychological Association.* Although there are many formatting styles, this template can serve as a basic guide in the organization and development of your ideas, thoughts, and references for papers required in your courses.

EXAMPLE 3

Example Skeleton Paper

A skeleton paper template can be used for all of your works in many online programs (Vain, 2008). All that needs to be changed is the content and the style of formatting that is required by your institution.

How To Use the Template

If you use a template, start each paper with the title and develop the headings by using the course assignment rubric. This creates a huge psychological edge that motivates you to write your paper and helps to dispel any writer's block (Monder, 2004).

FIGURE 7-1 Skeleton Template for Papers *(continued)*

EXAMPLE 4

Additional Bonus

Including a reference page in your template will help you to keep track of your references because you can add them as you type your paper. When you are finished writing your paper, your reference page is nearly done and is ready to be checked. The nice part of this bonus is that you know your reference page has all of your citations. You just need to alphabetize the list by the author's surname.

EXAMPLE 5

Why Templates Work

Research has shown that the drop in frustration levels of students writing papers for online programs is well documented when templates are used. In addition, students using templates have expressed a higher self-perception of happiness and relaxation (Douglas, 2006).

What Levels of Happiness Can Do

Increased happiness has been shown to improve grades, marriages, parent-child relationships, evaluations at work, and even skin tone (Adams, 2008). Imagine the possibilities.

Conclusion

By now, you should realize the phenomenal benefits of using a paper template for writing papers for your online educational programs. Good luck in all you do.

EXAMPLE 6

References

Adams, J. (2008). Peace be with you. *Journal of Helping Hands, 12*(2), 24-27.

Douglas, M. (2006). *A model for learning*. New York: Wooster House.

Monder, L. (2004). Writing in your own way. *Journal of Online Sources, 32*(14), 67-89.

Vain, I.M. (2008). *Tutorial of writing.* London: Westinghouse.

nearly complete in no time, allowing you time for editing and revisions. You can then use this completed paper as a template for future works. Your family, friends, and classmates will be amazed at the seemingly effortless manner in which you create excellent writing pieces time and time again.

Formatting and Style Guide

The overall goal of any formatting or editorial style is to facilitate clear and consistent writing that enhances reader comprehension (Cuddy, 2002). Although it may seem as though instructors are being needlessly demanding, most take very seriously their professional responsibility to ensure that graduating students have a basic, but solid, understanding of the formatting style that is used by the college, whether APA, MLA, AMA, or another. If a student is enrolled in a graduate-level program, it is likely that the individual will work in an academic environment at some point in his or her career. Without a doubt, an understanding of formatting style is essential in such a setting.

The following styles are used most often, although others could be required by some schools, programs, or journals:

- **American Psychological Association (APA)** style is taken from the *Publication Manual of the American Psychological Association* and is a popular style in schools and journals to cite sources within the social and behavioral sciences.
- **Modern Language Association (MLA)** style is used to write papers and cite sources within the liberal arts and humanities.
- **Chicago** style, which is comprised of two different reference styles, is used for the sciences (author-date system) and the humanities and social sciences (documentary-note style). It is based on the *Chicago Manual of Style.*
- **Turabian** style, a subset of Chicago style, is for college students to use for all subjects.
- **Council of Science Editors (CSE)** style is used in biology and other sciences and is described in *Scientific Style and Format: The CSE Manual for Authors, Editors, and Publishers.*
- **American Medical Association (AMA)** style, based on the *AMA Manual of Style,* is from the *Journal of the AMA* and is used in medicine, health, and the biological sciences.

There are numerous other formatting styles used by various journals and organizations that could be encountered in academic and/or postgraduate careers and settings. Information about each style is available, and usually easily accessible, in manuals, online, and from individual journals or associations. Almost all of these formatting styles have official Web sites and manuals that detail their rules and address frequently asked questions that greatly help novice writers as they begin to use the style. Most educational programs will advise the purchase of the necessary official style manual early in the course curriculum, if not at the very beginning. Buy the book and keep it handy. It will prove to be a worthwhile investment, and it will become an indispensable tool that you will use over and over again.

What Formatting Style Should I Use?

The decision of which formatting style to use is often predetermined by the specific educational institution, college, or journal. Although certain styles are generally used for specific disciplines, there is some overlap. Care should be taken to use the appropriate style for each specific purpose, as succeeding in a particular educational program or having an article accepted in a peer-reviewed academic journal is dependent on the correct and accurate use of the required style. Check the school's Web site or instructor notes, as well as course syllabi, for formatting requirements. Most journals have Web sites that have sections for authors, which include submission guidelines. Read articles in journals of interest to see what style is required.

The University of Phoenix, Walden University, and Case Western University all require APA formatting. Purdue's online campus uses MLA or APA, depending on the discipline. Check carefully and early to see which formatting style is required for a certain journal or school, and adhere to that style when writing and submitting work. This will save time and prevent the frustration and extra effort of reformatting the work later.

Why Is Formatting So Important?

If you are enrolled in an online educational program, chances are good that your time is at a premium. Maybe you have a full- or part-time job or have a family who depends on you, or both. You cannot afford to let the mere thought of writing a paper immobilize you. Even if you are able to start writing a paper, the formatting questions that will invariably arise can wreak havoc on a busy schedule. (The *Strategies to Deal With Expected Challenges* chapter in this book will help you to prioritize your needs during the time that you are enrolled in school.) Formatting tips can minimize distraction and the time wasted by stumbling blocks that have little to do with creative and scholarly abilities. Learning proper formatting from the onset of a program can help online students achieve their educational goals while living life, maintaining personal relationships, and succeeding at work.

The use of inaccurate style formatting can be detrimental to a cumulative grade point average. Point deductions for formatting errors can also be a great source of frustration and self-doubt for students. Most instructors demand that students use accurate style formatting in the hopes of fostering scholarly writing, not to be punitive. The more closely you adhere to the required formatting style, the easier your papers and manuscripts will be to understand, and the better your grades will be (Daniel & Onwuegbuzie, 2007).

Formatting is also very important when submitting work to peer-reviewed scholarly journals. The more prestigious the journal, the more important formatting becomes. Indeed, many book and journal editors will not even review a submission unless it is in the appropriate format, summarily rejecting the work if the usually clear and precise guidelines provided are not followed. However tedious it may seem, proper formatting is necessary for academic success and will become easier with time and practice.

Who Can Provide Formatting Assistance?

Take advantage of offers of help from instructors when they are extended. Most instructors are quite willing to answer formatting questions and provide advice about common errors in papers submitted by students. Remember, most instructors *will* deduct points for mistakes, although some instructors are more lenient than others. Take your formatting seriously and learn from your mistakes. After the first papers are graded and returned by a particular instructor, students will know the expectations of that instructor and can write accordingly. Pay careful attention to any early noted and/or recurrent problems, so that further point deductions can be avoided.

Formatting comes very easily to a handful of students in each online class or program. Some students have very few, if any, formatting point deductions. Those students are often quite willing to help classmates who are not as fortunate or studious, so do not hesitate to ask those peers for help. Asking a classmate can sometimes feel less threatening than emailing an instructor about a formatting issue, so go to the online student lounge and ask your questions. You could also individually email a few of the students who post lengthy discussion threads early and often. These overachievers are usually the ones who can format with ease or who may have had previous experience in another online program or course. If you ask nicely, someone might even look at your entire paper for you.

Formatting and Resources

Headings, the use of quotations, page set-ups, and reference citations are only a few of the areas that present problems for students who are trying to properly format a paper or manuscript. To minimize frustration, familiarize yourself with the many available resources that are found online, in software and manuals, or from your college or university, and choose what appeals to you.

Writing centers are offered by many online colleges and universities to help students improve their writing skills. These centers are generally accessible to students at no cost. If you plan on using these services, assignments must be completed early, as the turnaround time is often a week or longer. Although the reviewer may not be an expert, this process can provide an objective view of your work. Some writing centers will only look at the flow of the work, as well as major grammatical errors, and will not look at formatting issues, so check with your institution's writing center to see what they will do for you.

Web sites are also available through many colleges and universities that offer writing aids and formatting information to help students with writing assignments. Sometimes, students are required to have a log-in password to access these tools, but many sites are open to public viewing. These sites offer a wealth of information that can be quite helpful, especially for frequently asked formatting questions (see Table 7-1).

TABLE 7-1 A Sampling of Available Formatting Web Sites

Web Site	URL
APA Online	http://apastyle.apa.org
EasyBib Write Smarter	http://www.easybib.com
The OWL at Purdue	http://owl.english.purdue.edu/owl/resource/557/01
MLA Formatting & Style Guide	http://library.uncg.edu/depts/ref/qil/styles.asp
Citation Guides	
Long Island University Citation Style for Research Papers	http://www.liunet.edu/cwis/cwp/library/workshop/citation.htm
Bedford St. Martin's Research and Documentation Online	http://www.dianahacker.com/resdoc
A Research Guide for Students	http://www.aresearchguide.com/styleguides.html
Kent State Libraries & Media Services	http://www.library.kent.edu/page/10603
Walter E. Helmke Library Style Guides	http://www.lib.ipfw.edu/1063.0.html
PERRLA Your APA Home	http://www.perrla.com/Pages/1/2.aspx
Bergen Community College	http://www.bergen.edu/pages/2435.asp
Citing from Library Databases	
Doc Scribe's Guides to Research Style	http://www.docstyles.com
eazydatabase	http://www.eazypaper.com/products.cfm
Chapman University Style Guides	http://www1.chapman.edu/library/reference/styles.html
APA Style Essentials Vanguard University of Southern California	http://www.vanguard.edu/faculty/ddegelman/index.aspx?doc_id=796
APA Tips	http://academicwriting.suite101.com/article.cfm/apa_tips
Noodle Tools Software	http://www.noodletools.com
RefWorks–Cite & Manage Your Research	http://www.refworks.com
Son of Citation Machine–interactive tool	http://www.citationmachine.net

Talk to professionals in your field of study, and listen to the advice of others who have completed similar types of educational programs. Classmates who have experience with distance education can be rich sources of tips and tricks for novice online students and are usually quite willing to share. Reading peer-reviewed journals for style and formatting will also help you to write in a professional, appropriate, and academic manner.

An abundance of information in various forms is available for each of the formatting styles. The sheer amount of information can be overwhelming in itself. One need only to search the online bookstores, Web sites, or Amazon.com to see the many official and unofficial manuals, self-help books, and software downloads available on style formatting. Remember that you do not need to buy a lot of books or downloads, no matter how helpful they might seem. It is okay to use them if they work for you, but they are not necessary to succeed. The most useful manuals provide not only information on specific formatting issues, but also illustrations of actual reference pages or excerpts from a completed paper as examples of proper formatting. Most students do not need more than one manual, though, since additional help is readily available online or from other resources on schools' Web sites.

Read reviews of available formatting software and ask others, especially librarians and other students, about their experiences using specific software or downloads. Free demo downloads are often available; the demo version works for a limited time to let you see if you like the program. Some writers swear by the Web-based formatting services RefWorks and EndNote, which are often provided by academic university libraries to staff and students at no cost. Others use a free interactive Web tool, such as Citation Machine, with success. Some software that we use on a daily basis, such as Microsoft Word 2007, provides formatting aid for several styles. You may eventually find, however, that these programs are not as helpful to you as they seem at first, and will probably not do what you expect them to do.

To filter out the extraneous help out there, try a few low-cost or free ideas that might be beneficial. Find a simple reference sheet on the required formatting style that includes the basic rules of the style. Create it yourself from a manual or trusted Web site, or ask your instructor if your school provides one. Many Web sites offer such reference sheets that you can print and keep handy or bookmark for easy access.

Whatever resources you choose should work for you and should meet your unique technological aptitude, preference, and personal finance needs. Forewarned is forearmed. Overall, knowledge of and access to downloads, manuals, software, online help, and articles about formatting will make the online educational experience more rewarding and much less frustrating.

Formatting Tips and Tricks

You may want to save examples of the trickiest references or in-text formatting issues in a special, easily accessible file on your computer. In an online program that uses instructional

DVDs, for example, the citation for various lessons appearing on the DVDs can be a complicated one. Keeping that citation in a computer file and copying it whenever it is needed, changing only a few key words according to the lesson, can save much time and effort. You can also keep your skeleton paper template in the same file, along with your one-page cheat sheet of the basics. It is amazing how helpful such a small bit of simple organization can be. Really, any copy of an accurate reference list can serve as a guide for most papers. The more difficult formatting outliers—such as those electronic references with no date, author, or title, or the book with a different editor and author for each chapter, or those annoying secondary citations—can be addressed as needed with the style manual or another tool.

Formatting assistance has become more readily available over the past few years, from sources such as the latest office software programs and many online library Web sites. To that end, it is important to acquaint yourself with the word processing program on your computer that you use to write your papers, so that basic text formatting issues (how to make formatting happen using the software) do not confound style formatting issues (the formatting itself). The shortcuts that you can use (if you know that they are there) can remove a lot of the sting from making changes. For example, if you finish your paper and realize that you made a mistake in formatting throughout your work, you can make all the needed changes at once rather than changing every incidence individually. In addition to learning style formatting, it is equally important to know what your office software program can do for you as you write your papers or articles. It is worth the time to take the tutorials or a class on Microsoft Word (or whatever program you use) to learn what the program can do. At the same time, you will learn the style formatting capabilities of your software program. This added knowledge will undoubtedly make your writing days happier ones.

Common Mistakes in Formatting

There are a few common mistakes in formatting that become pet peeves of many online instructors and journal editors. Using a formatting checklist such as one of those at the end of this chapter while proofreading your work can help immensely in submitting error-free work, making it less likely that you will evoke the irritation of your instructor, who may be having a bad day after seeing the same mistakes in every paper he or she reads. (They are trying to help you learn to write effectively, but it is difficult to accept the point deductions if you are trying your best to comply).

The most common mistakes in formatting include the passive voice, incorrect heading levels, using quotations incorrectly, punctuation errors, wrong verb tenses, and, perhaps the most difficult, errors on the reference page and in the in-text citations (Daniel & Onwuegbuzie, 2007). The reference page usually requires the most attention, as it can be tedious and full of details (Gullen, 2008). The use of jargon can be another irritant to reviewers and readers, and should be avoided in most instances.

Proofreading can become your most effective tool, though if you have formatting issues, you will be so frazzled by the time you are finished with your paper that you may omit this important step out of sheer frustration and fatigue. The closer you get to the end of your educational program, the more likely you are to forgo proofreading. If you use a checklist, it might make this final check easier for you and help you to continue proofreading through to the end of your program.

Conclusion

The benefits of formatting scholarly works are indisputable for both the author and the reader. Formatting facilitates reader comprehension and provides the vital written consistency required in the academic setting. While formatting may induce writing anxiety in students who are already ill at ease with the writing process, numerous avenues for assistance with the formatting process are available at minimal or no cost to the users. The regular use of formatting may even result in improved grammatical structure, punctuation, and overall fluency and confidence in the writing process for students. With practice and patience, the use of formatting in scholarly compositions may help even the most timid writers develop exceptional writing skills.

Example Checklist for APA Formatting (American Psychological Association, 2010)*

______ Set margins as follows: one inch all around (top, bottom, left, right).

______ Make sure the title page (page one) includes the following: manuscript title, author(s) name, author (s) affiliation(s), running head and author note (if required). The title page should include uppercase and lowercase letters and the information should be centered on the page. (Make sure that you check with your institution and follow their recommendations.)

______ Verify that the font size is 12 point and the typeface is Times New Roman.

______ Include a concise, readable abstract on page two. An abstract may not be required for educational papers.

______ Make sure the text is double spaced and left aligned.

______ Check that paragraph indentation is five to seven spaces or 1/2 inch.

______ Set two spaces after periods at the end of sentences.

______ Verify that you have page numbers at the top right of every page beginning with the first page.

______ Make sure a running page header is on every page, is in all caps, is flush left at the top of the page, and does not include more than 50 characters (including spaces and punctuation).

______ Insert the title of the paper on the first page of text where the body of the manuscript is started.

______ Check that appropriate headings are used throughout the manuscript. Do not label the "introduction" as a heading.

______ For numbers under 10, use words; for 10 and higher, use numerals (exceptions do apply).

______ Check that in-text citations match the reference page.

______ Ensure that quotations of 40 words or more are set in block format, with no quotation marks, and each line is indented one-half an inch from the left margin.

______ Create a hanging indent in all lines after the first for each entry in the reference list.

______ Arrange the reference list entries alphabetically by author surname.

______ Proofread the text for spelling and grammatical errors.

*The 6th edition (copyright 2010) of the *Publication Manual of the American Psychological Association* was published during final review of this book. Given the timing of the publication of the 6th edition of the APA style manual, the rest of this book follows the styles outlined in the 5th edition (copyright 2001).

Formatting Checklist

______ Check to see which formatting style is recommended or required for your work before you begin and follow the guidelines carefully.

______ Purchase a formatting manual and keep it handy when writing.

______ Develop a quick-look reference sheet of frequently used formatting rules. Make your own or purchase one. This tool will prove to be invaluable.

______ Familiarize yourself with other formatting help and resources that can be found online, in software, and in hard copy, and choose what works best for you.

______ Use a template every time you write to get something down on paper quickly. This will supply the motivational support you need to complete the paper.

______ Use the course rubric or author guidelines for all of your work to ensure coverage of each requirement. Instructors and editors will see that you addressed each topic or guideline.

______ Save frequently used citations in a computer file so that they can be copied and pasted into new reference lists when needed.

______ Save all your corrected papers in a computer file for use as templates and for future formatting reference.

______ Take advantage of formatting help from instructors, librarians, classmates, and your school's writing center. They want to help you!

______ Use a formatting checklist for every paper that you write to ensure proper formatting.

References

American Psychological Association. (2001). *Publication manual of the American Psychological Association* (5th ed.). Washington, DC: Author.

American Psychological Association. (2010). *Publication manual of the American Psychological Association* (6th ed.). Washington, DC: Author.

Cuddy, C. M. (2002). Demystifying APA style. *Orthopaedic Nursing, 21*(5), 35–42. Retrieved October 24, 2008, from EBSCOhost database.

Daniel, L. G., & Onwuegbuzie, A. J. (2007). Editorial: Effective use of APA style in manuscript preparation. *Research in the Sciences, 14*(1), i–x.

Gullen, D. (2008). *APA tips. Suite101.com*. Retrieved November 10, 2008, from http://academicwriting.suite101.com/article.cfm/apa_tips

Nordquist, R. (2009). *About.com grammar and composition*. Retrieved December 13, 2008, from http://grammar.about.com/od/yourwriting/a/wblockquotes.htm

Chapter 8

Strategies to Maintain Health and Well-Being as a Student in the Online Learning Environment

Theresa A. Middleton Brosche[1]

Many online programs offer students tips, tools, and strategies to manage course workload, but very few offer students strategies to maintain health and well-being. Yet, maintaining health and well-being has been shown to enhance work productivity, increase mental performance, and foster emotional stability (Paton, 2005; U.S. Department of Health & Human Services, 2005; U.S. Department of Health & Human Services, 2008). This chapter will offer the following strategies to assist in maintaining health and well-being for students in the online learning environment:

- Ergonomic assessment and the desktop work space.
- Nutritional tips.
- An 8–10-minute movement routine.
- Stress-reduction techniques.

Ergonomic Assessment and the Desktop Work Space

Ergonomics is the science of designing a work space contoured to meet the needs of the worker (American Federation of Government Employees, 2009). Designing an ergonomically sound work space can enhance productivity and can minimize discomfort and fatigue of the head, neck, shoulders, eyes, hands, wrists, arms, and lower back. It can also reduce the risk of computer-related repetitive stress injuries such as carpal tunnel syndrome, back pain, neck pain, tennis elbow, temporomandibular joint (TMJ) dysfunction, shoulder impingement syndrome, and De Quervain's disease (Bonomo & Seidler, 1999), to name a few.

Creating an ergonomically sound work space, however, is often overlooked by students in the online learning environment because many individuals believe that ergonomics is applicable only to the work setting. Ergonomics is not only practical but essential for students in the online learning environment who sit for prolonged hours using repetitious

[1] The author of this chapter, Theresa A. Middleton Brosche, MSN, RN, CCRN, is an ACE certified personal trainer and an ACE certified lifestyle and weight management consultant.

movements of the muscles, ligaments, and joints in the shoulders, hands, wrists, forearms, and lower back.

Repetitive Stress Injuries Defined

Carpal tunnel syndrome—a syndrome of pain and discomfort that can extend from the forearm down to the wrist, hands, palms, and fingers and is caused by pressure placed on the median nerve, which is located on the palm side of the wrist (Mayo Clinic Staff, 2007).

Tennis elbow—pain and discomfort that can extend from the elbow down to the forearm and the wrist and is caused by inflammation or tiny tears in the tendons that attach the forearm muscle to the bone on the outside of the elbow (Mayo Clinic Staff, 2008a).

Temporomandibular joint (TMJ) dysfunction—pain or discomfort that can occur in the face, jaw, and neck and has been found to be associated with damaged, overworked, or misaligned cartilage, disks, and/or muscles around the temporomandibular joint (Mayo Clinic Staff, 2008b).

Shoulder impingement syndrome—pain, weakness, or loss of motion in the shoulder that can occur when there is a narrowing of the space between the acromion and the humeral head (Fongemie, Buss, & Rolnick, 1998).

De Quervain's disease—pain in the back of the thumb that can extend into the thumb or up the forearm and is caused by swollen tendons in the thumb (WebMD, 2009).

Head-to-Toe Assessment

A head-to-toe assessment is one approach used to systematically assess the student desktop work space to ensure the following: head, neck, shoulders, wrists, and arms are in proper alignment; eye strain is minimized; lower back is in neutral alignment and fully supported; upper legs and knees are properly angled; and feet are resting firmly on the floor. The goal of this assessment is creating a safe and comfortable work space that is ergonomically sound and minimizes or eliminates the risk of repetitive-stress injuries.

Head, Neck, and Shoulders

One of your goals should be to ensure proper alignment of your head, neck, and shoulders. Your head should be level, forward facing, and in line with your neck and spine. Your shoulders should be relaxed and pulled back and down. Avoid sustained flexion and sustained extension (Brooks, 2001) and keep all body parts relaxed and free of tension.

- Position the top of the monitor at eye level or 15 to 20 degrees horizontally below eye level (Occupational Safety & Health Administration [OSHA], 2008d). Bifocal wearers may need to lower the monitor (Department of Occupational Health and Safety [DOHS], n.d.).
- Use a sturdy document holder and position it off to the side but close to the monitor and at the same height and the same distance as the monitor (Comana, 2007; OSHA, 2008d). The document holder can also be positioned directly beneath the monitor.

- Position the chair directly under the desk so you can attain proper body alignment and your shoulders can rest comfortably against the upper aspect of the chair.
- Place frequently used items, including the keyboard, the mouse, and the monitor, in front of you and close to your body (Centers for Disease Control and Prevention [CDC], 2000, para. 3; OSHA, 2008a; OSHA, 2008b; OSHA, 2008c; OSHA, 2008e).
- Keep your head, neck, and shoulders relaxed.

Eyes

Another goal is to ensure that you minimize eye strain.

- Position the monitor approximately 20 to 36 inches (or about arm's length) from yourself (DOHS, n.d., para. 2; OSHA, 2008a; OSHA, 2008d).
- Minimize glare through the following measures:
  - Position the monitor at a right angle from windows or bright lights.
  - Shine desktop lights on documents rather than on the monitor.
  - Close window blinds, particularly if the light interferes in viewing the monitor screen.
  - Hang a large manila folder 2–3 inches over the monitor or tilt the monitor slightly forward to minimize glare from overhead lighting.
  - Purchase an antiglare monitor shield or filter, if necessary.
- Adjust the contrast and brightness on the monitor as needed.
- Keep the computer screen clean.
- Increase font size as needed.
- Change font color as needed.
- If you are purchasing a new computer, consider one with a larger screen.
- Keep your eyes moist, particularly in dry environments (OSHA, 2008d).
- Purchase glasses designed specifically for working at the computer if needed (CDC, 2000; OSHA, 2008d).
- Take a 3–5-minute eye break every 20–30 minutes (CDC, 2000) by looking at something other than the computer screen, by closing your eyes, or by placing your hands gently over your eyes.

Hands, Wrists, and Arms

Another ergonomic goal of your head-to-toe assessment should be to ensure proper position of your hands, wrists, and arms. Your wrists should be straight and in line with your forearms, and your forearms should be parallel to the floor. Your arms should hang comfortably at the sides of your body with your elbows bent at a 90–120-degree angle when your fingers are on the keyboard (OSHA, 2008b). Avoid positions that cause your elbows to flare out to the sides of the body or positions that cause your arms to rise up toward the head, thereby placing tension on your shoulders and neck.

- Armrests, if used, should be padded with soft material, have rounded edges wide enough to accommodate the width of the forearm, and should be properly angled to assist in supporting and maintaining proper body alignment (DOHS, n.d.). If the armrests interfere with maintaining proper body alignment, they should be removed from the chair.
- Position the keyboard so your wrists are straight and in line with your forearms, not flexed or extended. It may be necessary to adjust the table height, chair height, or keyboard angle, and/or to install a keyboard tray to attain this position. If you are sitting on a couch or in a bed, use an object such as a firm pillow to assist in maintaining this alignment (CDC, 2000).
- You can use wrist rests to assist in maintaining neutral alignment of your wrists; however, avoid using the wrist rest if neutral alignment cannot be attained and if the hands cannot move freely during typing. Ensure the wrist rest is soft but firm. A wrist rest made of gel-type material is ideal (OSHA, 2008f). Although there does not seem to be a true consensus of whether to use a wrist rest or not when taking rest intervals from typing, if you use one, be sure that only the heel or the palm of the hand rests on the wrist rest (Comana, 2007).
- Position the mouse the same height as the keyboard and use a mouse that allows unrestricted and free-flowing movements (CDC, 2000).
- Forearms, wrists, and elbows should rest lightly on the keyboard, the desk, the wrist rest, the mouse, and the armrest. Avoid resting on sharp-edged surfaces or surfaces that do not promote proper positioning.
- Pad sharp-edged surfaces.
- Adjust the sensitivity of the keys so keying requires only a gentle touch.
- Explore the use of devices that reduce wrist bending and gripping such as touch pads, touch screens, voice inputs, joysticks, trackballs, and alternate keyboards, to address specific physical needs or physical requirements (OSHA, 2008c, 2008e).

Lower Back (Lumbar Spine)

Another goal of the head-to-toe assessment is to ensure that the lower back is in neutral alignment and fully supported. Neutral alignment entails the following: the crown of your head is up, your shoulders are pulled back and down, your abdominal wall is engaged and held tight like a girdle, and, if you are in a seated position, the ischial tuberosity, or the sitz bones, serve as the base of support. You should attain neutral alignment in any type of position; that is, sitting, standing, declined sitting, reclined sitting, side lying, supine, or prone positions. Continually assess for neutral alignment, particularly when you begin to tire, because neutral alignment, also called neutral spinal posture, assists in protecting the integrity of the lumbar spine (Brooks, 2001).

- Fully support your lower back. If the desktop chair does not have full support to maintain the natural curvature of the lumbar spine, consider the use of a pillow, a towel, or a lumbar support pad.
- Use a chair that is appropriate for your hip size, is comfortably padded, has a waterfall front edge, a five-legged base with casters, and can recline at least 15 degrees (sitting in a slightly reclined position reduces compressive forces on the spine) (Cheatham, 2009; Comana, 2007, p. 13).
- Take a 3–5-minute minibreak every 20–30 minutes (CDC, 2000, para. 10) to change body position and to give your eyes a rest from looking at the monitor screen. Use a timer or alarm to serve as a reminder to take a break.
- Incorporate a strengthening and stretching exercise routine into your schedule on a regular basis.
- Consider the use of an exercise ball chair to assist in maintaining spinal alignment, balance, and circulation while seated at the desk. It is important to note, however, that you may need to limit the amount of time on the ball at the onset because there is no back support. As the body becomes accustomed to maintaining postural alignment, the time on the ball can be increased (Comana, 2007).

Upper Legs (Thighs) and Knees

Yet another goal of the head-to-toe assessment is to ensure proper angling of the upper legs and knees. To do this your hips should be slightly higher than your knees, and your upper legs should be parallel to the floor and 2–3 inches from the underside of the workstation. The angle of your knees should be approximately 90–110 degrees, and there should be 2–4 inches between the back of your knees and the edge of the seat (CDC, 2000, para. 6).

Part of correct body positioning stems from the height and angle of the furniture. The following measures might be helpful:

- Adjust the seat of the chair forward, backward, up, or down, if possible, to achieve proper positioning.
- Adjust the desk by raising it on concrete blocks or boards or cutting off the desk legs. The clearance under the desk should be approximately 20–28 inches high (Comana, 2007; OSHA, 2008a).
- Keep the area under the desk clean and uncluttered.

Feet

The head-to-toe assessment also includes a goal of ensuring that the feet rest firmly on the floor. Try the following to accomplish this goal:

- Place a footrest under your feet if, after adjusting the chair, your feet do not rest firmly on the floor.
- Make sure your feet are slightly forward of the hips.
- Flex and extend your feet and ankles and wiggle your toes frequently.
- Take a 5–10-minute maxibreak every 2 hours. This should include an activity such as a walk, a stretching routine, or a movement routine.

Nutritional Tips

Proper nutrition and hydration, combined with a regular exercise regimen, can enhance work productivity, increase mental performance, and foster emotional stability (Paton, 2005; U.S. Department of Health & Human Services, 2005; U.S. Department of Health & Human Services, 2008). Beginning or maintaining a sound nutritional and exercise regimen, however, is often placed at the bottom of a student's priority list. The ill effect of placing one's health and wellness low on the priority list may not be realized until years later, and to stress this point, many health and wellness professionals use the motto, "pay now or pay later."

To avoid the costs and stresses associated with unhealthy behavioral patterns that can arise weeks, months, or even years later, it is important to include simple, yet effective, strategies meeting the requirements of the mind, body, and spirit. Simple and practical nutritional tips include the following:

- *Hydration:* Fill a large jug with filtered water and keep the jug at the work space. Be sure the jug is cleaned before each use and the water is changed daily. The general recommendation is that women should consume 2.7 total liters (91 ounces) of fluid a day (total liters of fluid includes fluid from beverages and food), and men should consume 3.7 total liters (125 ounces) of fluid (Institute of Medicine, 2004, para. 2). Drinking eight 8-ounce glasses of water a day, also known as the 8 × 8 rule, can be used to assist in meeting the daily fluid recommendations (Mayo Clinic Staff, 2008c, para. 8).
- *Snacks:* Purchase healthy snacks to keep at the desk. Look for snacks that have the USDA organic seal. This seal certifies that the product follows certain guidelines and avoids the use of fertilizers, pesticides, sewage sludge, genetic modifications, and irradiation (United States Department of Agriculture, 2008). In addition, wash all fruits and vegetables before eating, watch portion size of all foods, and complement carbohydrates with a protein because carbo-

hydrates should not be eaten alone. Examples of handy, nutritious snacks include the following:

  - Whole grain crackers, toast, mini bagels with peanut butter or low-fat cream cheese
  - Pretzels, trail mix, baked chips (100-calorie packs can assist in controlling the serving size)
  - Low-fat cheese sticks or slices
  - Low-fat yogurt with a tablespoon of nuts (place food items that need to be chilled in a small lunch box or cooler)
  - Low-fat cottage cheese with a small amount of cinnamon (Khan, Safdar, Khan, Khattak, & Anderson, 2003)
  - Fruit
  - Sports nutrition bars and protein shakes. Avoid bars and shakes that are high in calories, sugar, sodium, and saturated fat. Do not assume that a sports nutrition label means that the product is healthy. Select a high-quality product that is free of fillers and sugar substitutes.
  - Vegetables such as cut-up carrots, celery, broccoli, and cauliflower served with hummus
  - Hard-boiled eggs
  - Rice cakes
  - Tofu
  - Soup (watch the amount of sodium in processed soups)
  - Unsweetened cereal
  - Oatmeal
  - Popcorn
- *Meals:* Prepare meals ahead of time.
  - Place prepared meals into small containers, and put them in the refrigerator or in the freezer.
  - Eat leftovers for lunch.
  - Prepare food in the morning, if you do not have leftovers. This is a great time management strategy so you can maximize your time during the day while you are working.
- *Frequency of eating:* Use an alarm as a reminder to eat. Nutritious meals that are smaller in portion size and eaten frequently throughout the day can curb your appetite, stabilize blood glucose levels, and give you the energy to complete the tasks at hand (Neithercott, 2008).

8–10-Minute Desktop Movement Routine

Prolonged sitting, prolonged viewing of the monitor screen, misaligned body postures, repetitive movements of the muscles, ligaments, and tendons, as well as compromised blood flow can lead to symptoms such as pain, numbness, tingling, burning, swelling, stiffness, decreased range of motion, decreased grip strength, headaches, double vision, blurred vision, and irritation of the eyes (Bonomo & Seidler, 1999; Comana, 2007). Incorporating a simple and practical desktop movement routine into your study schedule can help minimize these symptoms and also meet the requirements of the mind, body, and spirit, thereby maximizing productivity.

> **Caution**
>
> Before engaging in any movement-related routine be sure that you know your limitations and that you work within your ability. If you experience any pain or discomfort, stop the movement.

While this section of the chapter introduces an 8–10-minute desktop routine, there are also software programs, books, and online resources offering a wide range of desktop routines. Whatever routine you select, be sure that you perform a self-check to determine if your body is in neutral alignment, and maintain this alignment throughout the routine. Then, relax the mind and the body and engage the abdominal muscles. Engaging the abdominal muscles maintains postural alignment and provides a base of support.

Neutral Alignment

- The crown of your head is up and in line with your torso.
- Your chest is up and your shoulders are pulled back and down.
- Your abdominal wall is engaged and held tight like a girdle.
- Your spine is in neutral alignment and the natural curves in the neck and lower back area are maintained.
- If you are in the seated position, the ischial tuberosity, or the sitz bones, serve as the base of support.

Exercise 1: Engage the Abdominal Muscles

- While standing or sitting, place your hands above your hips and wrap them around your abdomen with the fingers of each hand pointing toward one another.
- Tighten your abdominal muscles by bringing them closer to the spine with each second. It is important to maintain the natural alignment and the natural curve of the spine when performing this movement.
- Breathe throughout the exercise.

- Perform this exercise over 10 seconds and repeat 3–5 times, 2–3 times a day. The goal is to create an automatic response so the abdominal muscles effectively engage without much thought or effort.

Exercise 2: Open and Close Your Mouth

- Open and close your mouth 6–10 times.

Exercise 3: Extend Your Fingers (Figure 8-1)

FIGURE 8-1

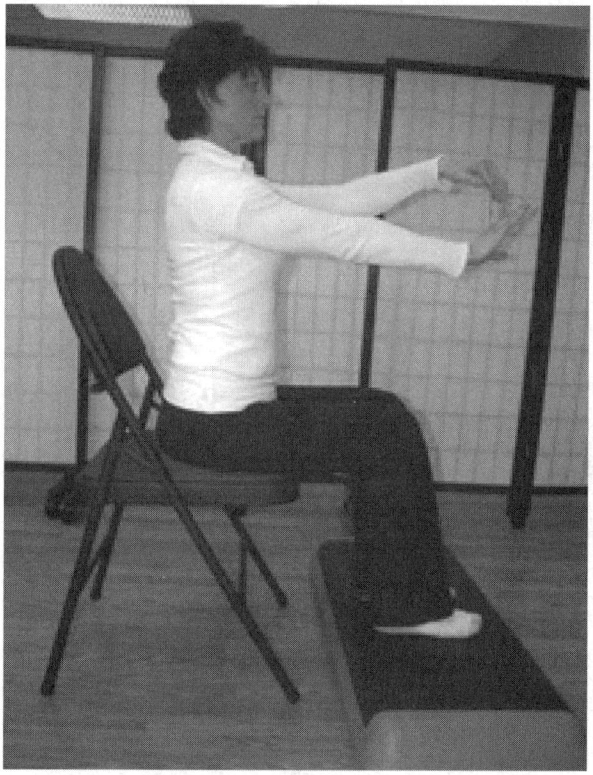

- Gently and slowly pull back each finger in succession and hold for a few seconds. Repeat this three times on each hand.

Exercise 4: Flex Your Wrists Forward (Figure 8-2)

FIGURE 8-2

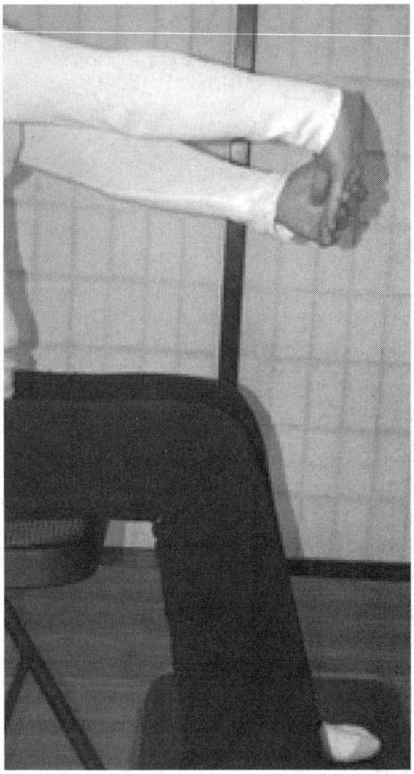

- Straighten one arm and turn the hand of that arm down so the fingers are facing the floor.
- Use the opposite hand and pull the fingers gently towards the body to feel a stretch in the forearm.
- Hold the stretch 10–30 seconds and then repeat it on the opposite side.

Exercise 5: Tip Your Wrists Down (Figure 8-3)

FIGURE 8-3

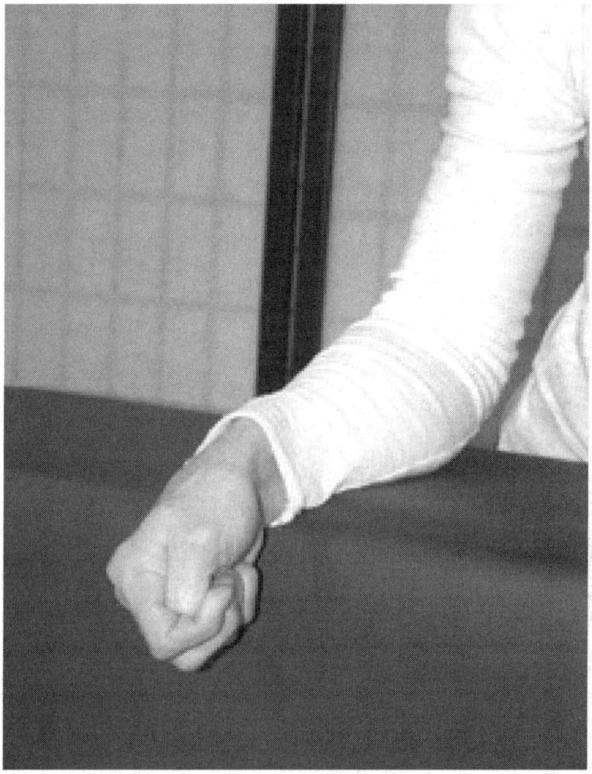

- Place your thumb on the palm of one hand and then close the fingers around the thumb.
- Turn the arm in, as if getting ready to use a hammer.
- While maintaining neutral alignment of the hand, wrist, and forearm, use your other hand to gently tip the wrist down to get a stretch in the tendon of the thumb. It may be easier to support the forearm on a soft surface when performing the stretch.

Exercise 6: Squeeze Your Shoulder Blades Together (Figure 8-4)

FIGURE 8-4

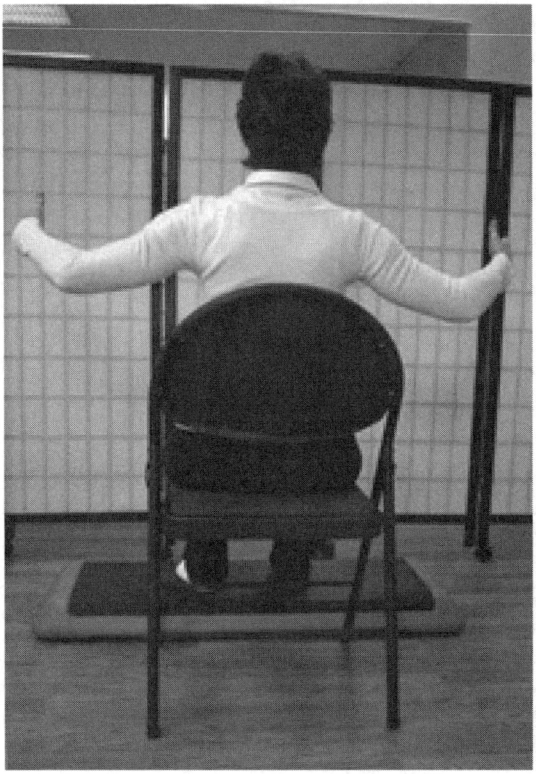

- Squeeze your shoulder blades together and flex your elbows 90 degrees.
- Slowly lean into the back of a chair or a wall to feel a stretch in your chest and the front of the shoulders.
- Hold the stretch for 5 to 7 seconds and repeat three to five times.

Exercise 7: Tilt Your Neck to the Side (Figure 8-5)

FIGURE 8-5

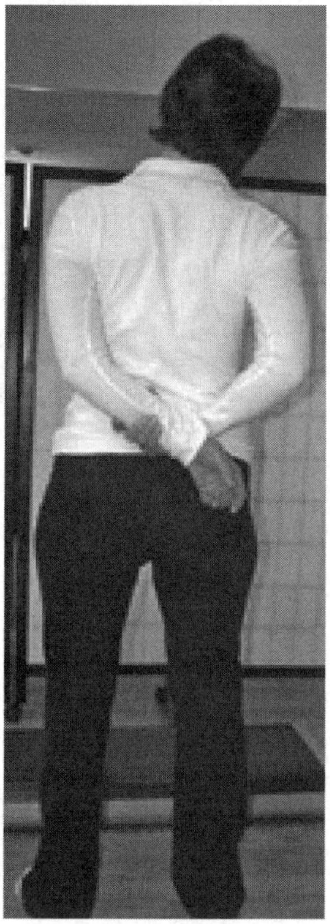

- Place one arm behind the lower part of your back with the palm of your hand facing outward.
- Tilt your head slightly to the opposite side of your body.
- Gently pull down on your arm behind the back of your body using the opposite hand.
- Hold the stretch for 10–30 seconds and repeat on the opposite side.

Exercise 8: Cross Your Legs (Figure 8-6)

FIGURE 8-6

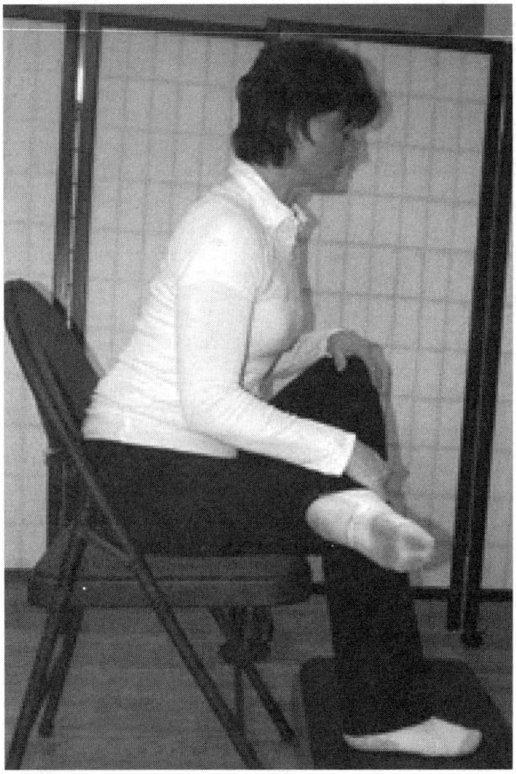

- Cross the ankle of one leg over the opposite knee.
- Keep your back straight and gently lean forward to feel a stretch in the buttocks and hips.
- Hold the stretch for 10–30 seconds and then repeat on the opposite side.

Exercise 9: Rotate Your Spine (Figure 8-7)

FIGURE 8-7

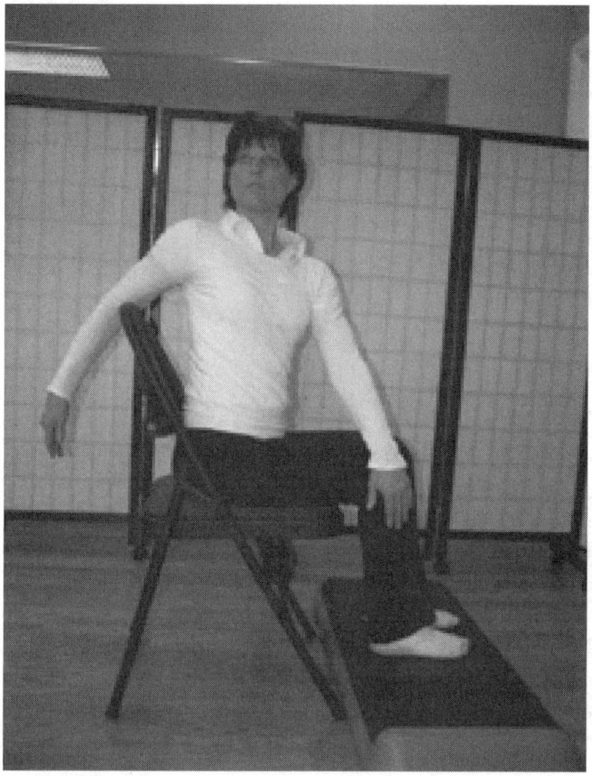

- With both feet on the floor, contract the abdominal muscles, keep your back straight and your hips straight and forward facing. Gently and comfortably twist your torso.
- Use your hands to gently deepen the stretch if so desired.
- Hold the stretch for 10–30 seconds and repeat on the opposite side.

Exercise 10: Lengthen Your Hip Flexors (Figure 8-8)

FIGURE 8-8

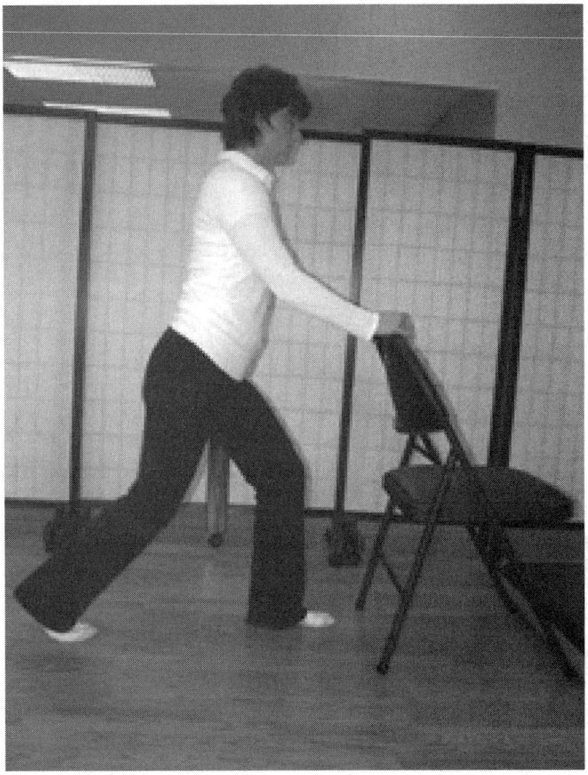

- Stand in a neutral posture and place one leg comfortably behind the other, keeping the knee of the front leg behind the top of the shoe/toes.
- Hold on to a sturdy, nonmovable object that can act as a base of support.
- Bend the knee of the leg that is behind the body and lower it until you feel a comfortable stretch in the hip flexor.
- Hold the stretch for 10–30 seconds and repeat on the opposite side.

Exercise 11: Flex and Extend Your Spine

- Get down on all fours with your wrists under your shoulders and your knees under your hips.
- Inhale. Drop your belly toward the ground and gaze slightly upward (Figure 8-9).

FIGURE 8-9

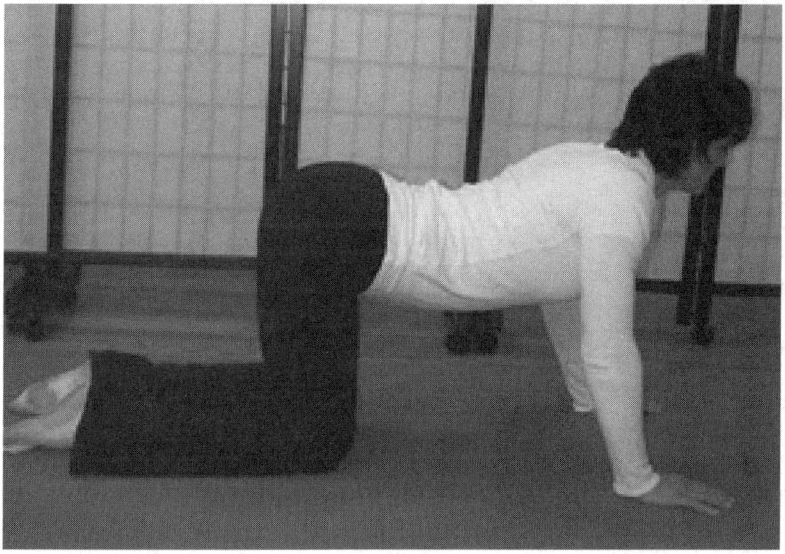

FIGURE 8-10

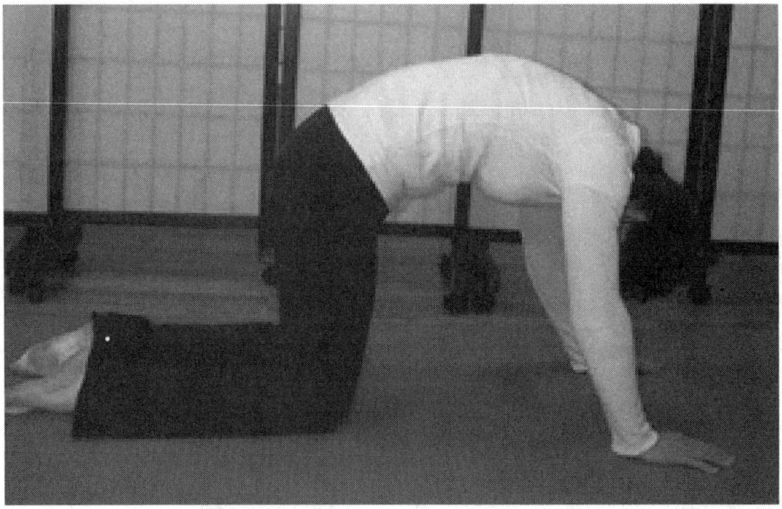

- Exhale. Hunch your back, drop your head, and gaze slightly down toward your navel (Figure 8-10).
- Perform the exercise 5–10 times slowly, inhaling and exhaling with each movement.

Stress-Reduction Techniques

Stress can lead to physical, emotional, and mental exhaustion, which may interfere with your ability in meeting deadlines, fulfilling obligations, and completing assignments. The use of simple, individualized measures can be used to calm the stress responses occurring while you are at work, at school, or at home. Some of these measures include the use of aromatherapy, music, walking, pictures, sayings, lighting, and breathing. Whatever technique is used, it is important that you choose something that is individualized to your needs and your preferences.

Aromatherapy

Aromatherapy uses pure essential oils to reduce anxiety (Tindale, 2007), improve concentration and mental clarity, increase energy, and/or elicit changes in mood. Incorporating aromatherapy into the work environment is easy because the essential oils used in aromatherapy can be found in candles, bath and shower gels, and lotions, or they can be inhaled through a diffuser. Some of the reported effects of the essential oils used in aromatherapy include the following (Kahn, 2007, p. 24):

- Ginger to stimulate energy and improve mental clarity.
- Pine to improve concentration.
- Geranium and rosemary to combat exhaustion, depression, tension, and mental fatigue.
- Lavender to reduce anxiety, promote relaxation, enhance arousal (Duan, Tashiro, Wu, Yambe, Wang, Sasaki, et al., 2007).

It is important to note that when choosing an essential oil, choose oils that are pure and have no additives. Artificial additives can cause side effects such as headaches, allergic reactions, and fatigue and be careful in the use of aromatherapy if you are pregnant because some of the essential oils are not recommended in pregnancy.

Music

Music has been shown to affect regions of the brain, eliciting physiological and emotional changes (Weinberger, 2004). Physiological changes can include changes in heart rate, blood pressure, and respiration, while emotional changes can include happiness, sadness, fear, tension, or euphoria (Weinberger). Before you decide to listen to music while you are working at your computer, ask yourself the following questions:

- Does music enhance your ability to work efficiently and effectively?
- Does music set the right mood for your studies?
- Do you feel relaxed or tense when listening to music?

Music and Work Productivity

I had been searching for a CD that I could play while working at my desk. The music I had tried when I was in school was distracting and did not enhance my work environment. During the writing of this chapter I was sent a CD by a professional musician from California called *Inner Aura*. The CD was designed to be used during yoga, massage therapy, and meditation; however, I used it while I worked at my desk. I found that the CD lowered my anxiety, decreased my heart rate and blood pressure, increased my work productivity, and complemented and enhanced my work environment.

Take a Walk

Walking on a regular basis can improve circulation, increase oxygen delivery, decrease anxiety, and increase work productivity. Removing yourself from a task that is overwhelming or has you overworked to take a walk can clear your head and help you feel more alert, refreshed, and ready to finish the project. Taking a walk can also bring about new ideas or a new outlook.

Walking and New Ideas

When I found myself reading the same sentence in my textbook or writing the same sentence several times for a class assignment, I would take a walk. During the walk I would think about the assignment and I would formulate new ideas and a new plan of attack. Although the walk may have only been 10 minutes long, I would return to my desk feeling more alert and full of new ideas.

Uplifting Pictures and Words

Uplifting pictures, words, sayings, and comments displayed in your work area can give you that extra boost to get you through the challenges you may face and the rough times you may experience. The student in the online learning environment who does not have face-to-face support can find this simple strategy an invaluable tool when times get tough. Sayings that worked for students in the past include the following:

"The only journey is the journey within."—Rainer Maria Rilke

"The distance is nothing; it is only the first step that is difficult." —Marie Anne du Deffand

"Heaven never helps the man who will not act."—Sophocles

"Knowing yourself is the beginning of all wisdom."—Aristotle

"If we did all the things we were capable of we would astound ourselves." —Thomas Edison

"Keep your eyes on the prize—the diploma!"—Desi Carter

"Suffering produces endurance, and endurance produces character, character produces expectation and hope."—Romans 5:2–4

"Only those who dare to fail greatly can ever achieve greatly."—Robert Kennedy

"Success consists of going from failure to failure without loss of enthusiasm." —Winston Churchill

"There are no gains without pains."—Ben Franklin

"The distance between insanity and genius is measured only by success." —Bruce Fierstein

Lighting

Working in a properly lit area helps create a pleasant atmosphere and a sense of well-being. To do this, take advantage of the natural light sources in your work environment. If the natural light is not adequate, use indirect lighting and avoid extremely bright lights. "Indirect lighting sends 90–100% of the light up to the ceiling and walls where it then reflects to the work area" (Industrial Accident Prevention Association, 2008, p. 3).

Relaxation Breathing

Consciously breathing in and out through your nose and/or mouth, in a slow and controlled fashion, "is the quickest way to experience the body's relaxation response" (Avery & Ryan, 2007, para. 3). In order for this strategy to be effective, select a breathing technique that works best for you and incorporate it into your daily regimen, particularly when you find you are in a situation causing undue stress, anxiety, or tension. An example of one breathing technique is as follows:

- Slowly inhale through your nose or mouth over 3–5 seconds. Your abdomen should expand outward but the rest of your body should stay relaxed.
- Then slowly exhale through your nose or mouth over 5–8 seconds as you continue to keep your body relaxed.
- Repeat several times.

Enjoy Life

Taking time to enjoy life may seem very difficult when you are a student. It is important, however, to make time to take care of yourself physically, mentally, and emotionally because no one else can do this for you. Stop and smell the roses, look at the beauty all around you, and spend time with the people who are important to you. Taking the time to maintain health and well-being as a student in the online learning environment is an investment that you will not regret.

Conclusion

This chapter presented practical, low-cost strategies to enhance work productivity, increase mental performance, and foster emotional stability for the student in the online learning environment. Although obviously not fail-proof, implementing some of these strategies into your daily regimen can assist in maintaining health and well-being so you can be productive in the classroom and enjoy your online learning experience.

Practical and Simple Workspace Checklist

If you are unable to check off any item, please refer to the "Head-to-Toe Assessment" section to see what modifications can be made to the workstation.

Head, Neck, and Shoulders

_______ Your head is level, forward facing, and in line with your neck and spine.

_______ Your neck is free from tension and in line with your head and spine.

_______ Your shoulders are free from tension and pulled back and down.

Eyes

_______ Eye strain is minimized.

Hands, Wrists, and Arms

_______ Your wrists are straight and in line with your forearms and do not flex backward or forward.

_______ Your forearms are parallel to the floor.

_______ Your arms hang comfortably at the sides of your body and do not raise up toward your head.

_______ Your elbows are bent at a 90–120-degree angle when your fingers are on the keyboard, and your elbows do not flare out to the sides of the body.

Lower Back

_______ Your lower back is in neutral alignment and is fully supported.

Upper Legs and Knees

_______ Your upper legs are parallel to the floor and 2–3 inches from the underside of the workstation.

_______ The angle of your knees is approximately 90–110 degrees, and there is 2–4 inches from the back of your knees and the edge of the seat.

_______ Your hips are slightly higher than your knees.

Feet

_______ Your feet rest firmly on the floor.

References

American Federation of Government Employees. (2009). *Ergonomics.* Retrieved January 27, 2009, from http://www.afge.org/Index.cfm?Page=Ergonomics

Avery, A., & Ryan, M. J. (2007). Breathe easier. *Health, 21*(4), 163. Retrieved February, 1, 2009 from EBSCO database.

Bonomo, P., & Seidler, D. (1999). *ErgAerobics.* New York: ErgAerobics, Inc.

Brooks, D. (2001). *Effective strength training: Analysis and technique for upper-body, lower-body, and trunk exercises.* Champaign, IL: Human Kinetics.

Centers for Disease Control and Prevention (CDC). (2000). *Computer workstation ergonomics.* Retrieved September 30, 2008, from http://www.cdc.gov/od/ohs/Ergonomics/compergo.htm

Cheatham, S. (2009). Training the middle-aged back. *ACE Certified News, 15*(1), 6–8.

Comana, F. (2007). Expand your professional services with ergonomic evaluations. *ACE Certified News, 13*(1), 11–13, 24.

Department of Occupational Health and Safety (DOHS). (n.d.). *Ergonomics for computer workstations.* Retrieved September 30, 2008, from http://dohs.ors.od.nih.gov/ergo_computers.htm

Duan, X., Tashiro, M., Wu, D., Yambe, T., Wang, Q., Sasaki, T., et al. (2007). Autonomic nervous function and localization of cerebral activity during lavender aromatic immersion. *Technology and Health Care, 15*(2), 69–78. Retrieved February 1, 2009, from EBSCO database.

Fongemie, A. E., Buss, D. D., & Rolnick, S. J. (1998). Management of shoulder impingement syndrome and rotator cuff tears. *American Family Physician, 57*(4), 667–674, 680–682. Retrieved February 7, 2009, from http://www.aafp.org/afp/980215ap/fongemie.html

Industrial Accident Prevention Association. (2008). *Lighting at work.* Retrieved February 7, 2009, from http://www.iapa.ca/pdf/lightin.pdf

Institute of Medicine. (2004). *Dietary reference intakes: Water, potassium, sodium, chloride, and sulfate.* Available from http://www.iom.edu/?id=54343

Kahn, S. (2007). Does your energy need a boost? *Better Nutrition, 69*(4), 24–25. Retrieved February 6, 2009, from ProQuest Nursing & Allied Health database.

Khan, A., Safdar, M., Khan, M. M. A., Khattak, K. N., & Anderson, R. A. (2003). Cinnamon improves glucose and lipids of people with type 2 diabetes. *Diabetes Care, 26*(12), 3215–3218. Retrieved February 6, 2009, from http://care.diabetesjournals.org/cgi/reprint/26/12/3215

Mayo Clinic Staff. (2007). *Carpal tunnel syndrome.* Retrieved February 7, 2009, from http://www.mayoclinic.com/health/carpal-tunnel-syndrome/DS00326/DSECTION=symptoms

Mayo Clinic Staff. (2008a). *Tennis elbow.* Retrieved February 7, 2009, from http://www.mayoclinic.com/health/tennis-elbow/DS00469/DSECTION=causes

Mayo Clinic Staff. (2008b). *TMJ disorders.* Retrieved February 7, 2009, from http://www.mayoclinic.com/print/tmj-disorders/DS00355/DSECTION=all&METHOD=print

Mayo Clinic Staff. (2008c). *Water: How much should you drink every day?* Retrieved January 31, 2009, from http://www.mayoclinic.com/health/water/NU00283

Neithercott, T. (2008). The art of grazing. *Diabetes Forecast, 61*(10), 45–48. Retrieved February 6, 2009, from ProQuest Nursing & Allied Health Source database.

Occupational Safety & Health Administration (OSHA). (2008a). *Desks.* Retrieved January 31, 2009, from http://www.osha.gov/SLTC/etools/computerworkstations/components_desk.html

Occupational Safety & Health Administration (OSHA). (2008b). *Good working positions.* Retrieved January 31, 2009, from http://www.osha.gov/SLTC/etools/computerworkstations/positions.html

Occupational Safety & Health Administration (OSHA). (2008c). *Keyboards.* Retrieved January 31, 2009, from http://www.osha.gov/SLTC/etools/computerworkstations/components_keyboards.html

Occupational Safety & Health Administration (OSHA). (2008d). *Monitors.* Retrieved January 31, 2009, from http://www.osha.gov/SLTC/etools/computerworkstations/components_monitors.html

Occupational Safety & Health Administration (OSHA). (2008e). *Pointer/mouse.* Retrieved January 31, 2009, from http://www.osha.gov/SLTC/etools/computerworkstations/components_pointers.html#

Occupational Safety & Health Administration (OSHA). (2008f). *Wrist/palm supports.* Retrieved January 31, 2009, from http://www.osha.gov/SLTC/etools/computerworkstations/components_wrist_rests.html

Paton, N. (2005). Big name firms use high-profile campaigns to get staff healthier. *Occupational Health.* Retrieved January 31, 2009, from ProQuest Nursing & Allied Health Source database.

Tindale, R. (2007). Aromatherapy. *Emergency Nurse, 15*(6), 4–5. Retrieved February 6, 2009, from HealthSource Nursing/Academic Edition database.

United States Department of Agriculture. Agriculture Marketing Service. (2008). *National organic program.* Retrieved January 28, 2009, from http://www.ams.usda.gov/nop

United States Department of Health & Human Services. (2005). *Being healthy matters to you.* Retrieved February 2, 2009, from http://www.health.gov/dietaryguidelines/dga2005/healthieryou/html/chapter3.html

United States Department of Health & Human Services. (2008). *Physical activity has many health benefits.* Retrieved February 2, 2009, from http://www.health.gov/paguidelines/guidelines/chapter2.aspx

WebMD. (2009). *Arthritis: de Quervain's disease information.* Retrieved February 7, 2009, from http://www.webmd.com/rheumatoid-arthritis/de-quervains-disease

Weinberger, N. M. (2004). Music and the brain. *Scientific American, 291*(5), 88–95. Retrieved February 1, 2009, from EBSCO database.

Chapter 9

Communicating by Computer

Elizabeth L. Pratt

Scholarly communication is crucial for student success in the online learning environment. This dialogue involves the proper use of spelling, grammar, and punctuation with a thorough understanding of the necessities of online communication. The multitude of abbreviated forms of communication, such as text messaging, instant messaging, and twittering, have severely impacted the ability of individuals to communicate properly and effectively. This chapter will discuss the rules of engaging in electronic communication with both peers and faculty. Strategies to assist in implementing these rules into your online coursework will also be discussed in order to assist in minimizing misunderstandings and conflicts that can lead to a loss of points from formatting errors.

Correct Online Communication

Upon entering the world of online communication, it is important to be patient with yourself and others, as there will often be varying levels of experience with electronic forms of communication. There will also inevitably be different styles of communicating through the electronic format. Regardless, it is crucial to be able to communicate the right message, at the right time, to the right person, using the right format.

Netiquette

While everyone thinks and communicates in a unique way, there are certain rules that apply to everyone when communicating by computer. This set of rules is referred to as "netiquette." Netiquette is heavily influenced by the community of users and the circumstances surrounding the online communication (Aranda, 2007). In the case of online learning, netiquette will generally be established by the school or the instructor teaching the course. It is important to check to see if your school has listed any specific guidelines or formats that must be followed in order to avoid penalty for doing something considered incorrect or improper.

There are many netiquette guidelines that are of a common sense nature, as manners matter even on the computer. If you question whether something you write could be misleading, misread, or could cause interpersonal conflict, you may want to take a closer look at how you worded your idea. Consider asking for feedback from a faculty member or offer clarification with additional information if you have already hit the Send button. These strategies will demonstrate a respect for your fellow peers and faculty, as well as a willingness to learn more effective ways of communicating your thoughts and ideas.

All Caps, Font Style and Color, and the Use of Icons

A major consideration, and one paramount to setting the right tone with any online communication, is the use of all capital letters. Inexperienced users may feel that this typing strategy can make the message easier to read. In the online world, however, it is considered the equivalent of yelling at someone. Typing in all capital letters can lead to misunderstandings and conflict, and it can also make it difficult for the reader to follow what is being communicated (Aranda, 2007). In addition, a message can appear blurred and unreadable because the words seem to run together, particularly for those individuals with vision problems.

> **All Caps Email From a Student**
>
> MRS. PRATT, I WILL MISS CLASS ON MONDAY DUE TO A FUNERAL. IS THERE ANY WAY THAT I CAN SUBMIT MY ASSIGNMENT 1 DAY LATE? I NEED YOU TO LET ME KNOW AS SOON AS POSSIBLE. IF I DON'T HEAR FROM YOU BY 3 PM, I WILL CALL YOUR OFFICE OR CHECK WITH YOU AGAIN IN THE MORNING. I APPRECIATE YOUR UNDERSTANDING. THANK YOU.

Another consideration is the style and color of the font. Netiquette dictates that you use a font that is easy to read. For example, The lazy cow jumped over the moon appears here in Times New Roman font, and here, *The lazy cow jumped over the moon* is in Freestyle Script. Although both examples are written in a font size of 12 points, the first example is clearly much easier to read than the latter. Netiquette also dictates that if you use a font color other than black, it should be pleasing to the eye and able to be read by anyone. The use of different font colors is usually for emphasis only. Including color in coursework could result in the loss of points if not approved by the faculty prior to use. In addition, people who are color blind can have a hard time distinguishing red from green and blue from yellow (Hoffman, 1999).

A final consideration is the use of emoticons. An emoticon, as it refers to e-communication, is an abbreviation or a visual icon used to convey an emotion, such as LOL (laughing out loud) or ☺ to indicate humor or amusement. These inserts are unacceptable in any formal communication, including postings in the online classroom and emails related to academia. They can detract from the message you are trying to convey, can slow the reader down, or can be interpreted as annoying, irritating, rude, or distracting to some people.

Delivery and Read Receipts

Delivery receipts and read receipts are methods of proof that your email or homework assignment was received by the recipient's computer (delivery receipt) and/or opened by the recipient (read receipt). Similar to the U.S. Postal Service's signature required method of mail delivery, these receipts confirm that the assignment, document, or message was delivered to the right person at the right time. This is especially important when a student could lose points by submitting an assignment late.

Not every computer system or email client has the read receipt and delivery receipt functions, but for those that do, it is a good idea to utilize it, particularly when taking classes in the online learning environment. To maximize the usage of these receipts, place them in a specific folder in your email system and save the folder until you have completed the course and are confident that the receipts will no longer be needed.

> **Useful Proof That an Assignment Was Delivered on Time**
>
> When I was a student in an online master's program, a faculty member subtracted two points from an assignment that she believed had been submitted late. Since I had saved the delivery receipt, I was able to prove to her that I had, in fact, submitted my work on time and the two points were added back to my grade.

Threaded Discussion

A threaded discussion is a group of messages or postings related to a specific topic. Threaded discussions are an important component in the online learning environment, as they encourage and foster communication among students and faculty. This type of communication can lead to a healthy exchange of ideas and thoughts, or a discussion of information found in required readings.

Generally, the topic of the initial thread and the requirements for responses are determined by the faculty member who is teaching the course. Common rules for engaging in threaded discussion include the following:

- It is not necessary to respond to each new thread, unless otherwise specified as a course requirement.
- Include a concise heading to make it clear what your topic or response is about.
- Respond to the thread that has already been started instead of beginning a new thread altogether. Otherwise, it can be very confusing for others trying to figure out which responses belong to which thread.
- Stay on topic. A threaded discussion is not the place to present your personal agenda or your political beliefs.
- Do not use terms that are inaccurate or inappropriate. No one wants to have to read between the lines in order to figure out what your posting is about. These postings can also cause serious problems with your grade and your overall chances of successfully completing the course.

Spam

Spam is considered unsolicited junk email (Federal Trade Commission, 2008). When taking an online course, you will have access to many email addresses, both from peers and from faculty. Some of these addresses will be home addresses, while others will be work addresses. Sending jokes, pictures, and funny messages to these email addresses is considered spamming and is unwelcome. Not only does the recipient need to spend time going through and deleting all of these emails, but you could be sending the emails to a work address where an individual has signed a formal agreement that computer usage is for work purposes only. Your spam would violate that agreement, and this could lead to a verbal warning or even termination of that individual. In addition, although you may not consider an email to be offensive, it may be offensive to others. The basic rule for spamming is that you should not use an email address in such a manner without the express knowledge or consent of your peers and faculty. Also keep in mind that when you forward a message that includes personal email addresses, you are sending out private information without consent, which is a big faux pas.

Flaming

Flaming is the practice of saying in print what you feel, without regard to tact or the feelings of others (The Virginia Adult Learning Resource Center, 2007). Flaming wars begin when individuals start openly criticizing one another in the online environment. Emotional responses should be avoided at all times in your postings and emails. Prevent flaming by using a professional and respectful atmosphere in all online communication.

Email Tone

Online communication needs to be considerate and respectful of your peers and faculty. While no one hears your posting, the words alone convey a tone. Express respect, even when disagreeing or presenting a differing view. Common rules for verifying a proper email tone include the following:

- After completing your email or assignment, reread the material.
- If you are concerned about the possibility of an improper tone, ask someone else (e.g., family member, friend, colleague) to review it, specifically evaluating for any problems with tone. Others usually hear the tone you may have missed. An objective review will lessen the chance for conflict.
- As previously mentioned, do not use all caps for emphasis. Use an exclamation point, italics, or a bold font instead.

Looking Good Online

Avoiding Misinterpretation

A large concern in online communication is the avoidance of misinterpretation of words and/or thoughts. It is easy to forget that we are dealing with real humans through a monitor devoid of emotion, facial expression, and voice inflection. With online communication, the written word is your only representation, and it must be presented with tact and sensitivity. Avoid conflict by not giving your opinion (unless asked for), but state and interpret the facts only. If you would not say something to a person face to face, then you should not express it in writing (Shay, 2008).

When presenting a different view, express your thoughts in a positive manner. Avoid words associated with negative connotations, such as *don't*, *won't*, *can't*, *no*, *hate*, and *not*. Avoid using words associated with anger, shame, guilt, fear, or sadness. In general, our vocabulary contains more negative words than positive ones. Making your communication positive will require effort and specific attention to the words you choose (Schrauf, 2005).

In all online communication, be concise and to the point. Long-windedness frustrates your reader and is likely to lead to a misinterpretation of words and a lack of interest on the part of the reader. Initially use short, plain sentences until it has been established that English is the primary language of your peers and faculty. Avoid using words that you do not fully understand yourself. For questions about instructions regarding an assignment, ask your faculty member prior to the deadline in order to avoid a misunderstanding that may ultimately affect your grade.

Conveying Respect in Your Emails

An email from a student to a faculty member said, "Hey, you told me to tell you when I wasn't going to be in class so I'm telling you that I won't be there tomorrow." There is no salutation addressing the faculty member, nor does the student sign the email. In this case, determining the sender required checking the properties link of the email address. This was both time-consuming and frustrating for the recipient. The student showed a lack of respect by failing to correctly address the faculty. Instead of a casual greeting, this student should have started with a proper greeting to the faculty prior to the body of the email.

Conveying Respect

Demonstrate respect with written communication simply by addressing a person by his or her proper name. Specifically, when emailing faculty members, know whether to address them as Mr., Mrs., Ms., or Dr. Use of the proper title confers respect for the person's position. For peers, addressing by first names may or may not be appropriate. Make sure to spell names correctly.

When concluding your email or posting, close with your name. Specifically for emails, include a signature line containing your full name and further contact information (e.g., email address, phone number, and/or home or school address). A permanent signature is an option that can be added to emails. Consult your operating guide to find specific instructions.

For online classes, verify when faculty is available via email. Consider asking the following:

- Is email checked several times a day or just once every 24 hours?
- Is email checked on the weekend?
- Will faculty notify students when they are not going to be reachable by email?
- How long should a student wait for a response from an initial email before attempting to contact the faculty member again?

Grammar and Spelling Issues

Grammar and spelling errors are common mistakes in online communication. Utilizing the computer's grammar and spell checks will not guarantee that everything is correct. Grammar check does not catch common mistakes, such as typing "no" instead of "now." Set your computer to capitalize words as needed ("I" instead of "i"). Specifically check for these errors when reviewing your work. Make an effort to read everything at least twice prior to sending or submitting.

Email with Attitude

A student sent an email after group assignments were announced. It said:

> Mrs. Pratt, I really don't understand why you didn't put me in the group with the other students like I specifically asked you to do. I guess you don't care that I will have to meet with them online at a time that really isn't convenient for me in order to get the group project done.
>
> A follow-up email arrived about 15 minutes later, saying,
>
> Mrs. Pratt, I am so sorry for sending my previous email. I was taking my frustration out on you after having a fight with my soon-to-be ex-husband about some childcare issues, so that I can continue to work and go to school. I apologize for the other email and promise to never send another email while I'm angry. Thank you.

Attitude in Online Communication

Avoid sending or writing an email or a posting when you are tired, angry, ill, or having a bad day. Mistakes are easily overlooked and things can be said that may later have serious consequences (Shay, 2008). If you do make the unfortunate mistake of posting or sending an email with improper content, acknowledge your mistake as soon as possible.

Presenting Different Views

To present a differing view, make sure to use factually based evidence. Stay on topic. Avoid name calling or arguing over who is right and wrong. Before responding to a heated email or discussion posting, cool off. Avoid posting thoughts about subjects unrelated to the required elements. Read postings carefully. Ask questions to clarify, rather than attack statements of others. Let others post comments before you join in again if conflict arises, or ask the faculty member to intercede as a moderator (The Virginia Adult Learning Resource Center, 2007). Open yourself up to the thoughts of others for the benefit of learning before condemning them as wrong based on your initial reaction.

If you want to have a personal debate regarding information from a posting, invite your peer to email you personally, or visit a chat room to avoid subjecting everyone else to your debate. If he or she refuses, stop. Avoid developing a reputation as someone who argues over everything, giving you a negative position in the class. Your peers and faculty will notice the argumentative individuals and will stay away from interactions with them to avoid any chance of conflict.

Sending the Wrong Message: Common Pitfalls

Emails are frequently sent, forwarded, or replied to the wrong person. You are responsible for double checking the name(s) in the Send To box. The most common mistake in regards to email is forwarding to or replying to the wrong person. Everyone can blind carbon copy (BCC) an email. This prevents recipients from seeing who else received the same email. Emails can be forwarded without your permission to unknown individuals. A good rule of thumb is that if you are not willing to see it again, you should not put it into writing. In this day of technology, anything that you transmit electronically can be brought back around to you again, even years in the future.

Many email systems store email addresses frequently used in an address book. Entering "Jane" will bring up every Jane you have ever communicated with via email. When writing an email, names can pop up and be selected for use with one click over the right name. Email systems should not be set up to send emails using a first name only, but should require validation of the intended recipient. This can generally be accomplished by always entering both a first and a last name for your contacts (e.g., John Doe), or a specific title, such as Nurse Jane.

Faculty frequently use email as the method of choice for transmitting course information. Students should check their email on a regular basis. Based on the course and faculty, this may be required daily or just every few days. Failing to check email on a regular basis can have serious consequences. Avoid assuming that you know what information is in an email based on title alone. Read each email in its entirety prior to deleting or moving it to an assigned folder. Keep copies of your email correspondence with your peers and faculty in case the correspondence is needed again during the course. Others prefer to keep a copy of every email and posting until the entire program of study has been completed.

Things You Should Never Say

Avoid both insinuating a threat and/or stating it outright. Also avoid the use of potentially offensive language. Putting a threat in writing can be cause for genuine concern of your

> **Addressing Problem Areas**
>
> Student No. 1 only posted two sentences for the new posting of the week. It was obvious to everyone that her posting was incomplete. Instead of a private email, student No. 2 decided to publicly chastise student No. 1 for leaving off part of her posting. This led to several unpleasant posted interactions between the two students. At that point, the faculty member stepped in to let student No. 2 know that his manner in handling the entire situation had not been appropriate. The faculty member had already been in contact with student No. 1 via a private email to discuss the problem with the posting. However, the damage between the two students was already done, since student No. 2 clearly felt that he was in charge of correcting his peers.

peers and the faculty with possible legal implications for you. Direct confrontation may also be taken as a threat. A threat made on the Internet can be traced back to you and your physical location by the authorities. All of these actions could possibly lead to criminal charges. If you personally feel threatened, always notify the appropriate individuals as listed in your educational institution's policy.

Faculty members are the ones responsible for addressing a student's problem areas. It is not one student's responsibility to correct another, and doing so will only foster resentment from his or her peers. If there is a mistake, as in a posting, that has been obviously overlooked, and you feel that you must address it, do so politely, and preferably by a private email rather than public confrontation (Shay, 2008).

Avoid posting comments that do not contribute to the overall discussion in progress. Post meaningful input, saving one-word responses for face-to-face interactions. The same applies to two- or three-word phrases such as "I agree," "Great job," or "Well said." These short phrases add to the amount of material to be read by your fellow students, without any significant contribution to the ongoing discussion. Be open to constructive criticism regarding your postings without taking offense.

Handling Conflict

If you have a conflict with a faculty member, follow the educational institution's chain of command. If you cannot find this information in the course syllabus, contact your advisor or educational facility. If two students cannot resolve a conflict peacefully on their own, it may be time for faculty involvement. Occasionally, students will simply have to agree to disagree in order to resolve a conflict. Avoid using a demanding tone to tell the faculty member how you feel the situation should be handled. Also avoid making assumptions based on your feelings alone.

Apologizing

Apologizing is the quickest way to avoid hurt feelings, poor attitudes, and/or conflict with both your peers and faculty. Apologize as soon as you realize that you have made an erroneous assumption, or have made an inappropriate comment. This is not the time to be

Conflict with a Faculty Member

The following email was received by a faculty member from a student who was unhappy with the group he had been assigned to:

> I was online getting directions for our project and noticed that you decided to put me in a group that is inconvenient for me. I have tried to be very nice and professional to everyone so far this semester. I sent you a previous email telling you when I was and was not working and I asked you specifically to not put me in the group that was assigned to meet on certain days and times. You replied that you would do the best you could to avoid any conflict with my work schedule. Now, since you put me in the wrong group, I am going to have to adjust my work schedule, as I still need to provide for my family while I am in school! I feel as if this is some sort of harassment towards me. There are several other people who could be in this group and not have to worry about work conflicts. I know because I've asked them and when I suggested this to you, I was told that the groups were assigned for a reason. I am going to do my very best, but I really find what I was told and what has happened to be very dishonest. Even in this email I have been nice, honest, and professional. Whatever I have done to make you dislike me, just let me know, and I am sorry for it. I will do my best no matter how people feel about me.

The faculty member perceived this email as filled with angry tones and untrue accusations of unfair treatment. The student was informed that there were many reasons he had been assigned to the group, even though he seemed to feel that the group work would interfere with his work responsibilities. The student was reminded that he could request his group to change meeting times. The dates and times listed in the assignment were only suggestions. After further discussion with the faculty member and difficulties with working in the assigned group, the student dropped the course, citing unfair treatment by the faculty and his peers.

bullheaded. Do not wait for the other person to apologize. You will be wasting valuable learning time by concentrating your efforts on being offended, as opposed to moving on with your learning. Take the first step to correct the issue and proceed with your learning on a positive note. When you find yourself needing to apologize, make it brief and to the point. Don't try to impress; apologize and move on.

Student Lounge and Communication

The student lounge in the online learning environment is where students are often asked to introduce themselves to their classmates, providing such information as physical location, educational background, and other information in order to personalize encounters with both peers and faculty. The type of information requested in the student

Conflict via Email

I had a student who was not passing my online course. Over the course of half the semester, I made at least six attempts via email and three attempts via phone to discuss with her the reason for her poor assignment submissions and to give her directions about things she needed to work on in order to improve her grades. After 2 weeks had passed with no submission of an assignment, I sent an email to the student, informing her that she was being dropped from the course according to university protocol for lack of participation as required by the grading rubric. The following email from the student contains the mistakes in spelling/grammar as received [boldface added to reinforce the errors].

> Mrs. Pratt, I am just now **being able** to open my email because my home computer has been down for the last week, but Greg told me that he sent in my assignment for me the **Wendesday** before Spring Break. **now** what happened to it I don't know, **bit** it was sent and you can check with him if you think it is false. I can **have** you the number and if you dropped me from the class because I didn't send in assignments I am not paying for the class and **i** need to be **reimburse** for the class because I sent my part and I **ask** him to send it and he told me he sent it. I **dont** think I should be dropped **for** the class because he **didnt** send it and I will be calling your boss about this first thing Monday morning. I have **ran around** and got all this **stuff together turned** my work **in and work**, took care of a child **and you going** to drop me over an assignment **cause** you want to. If **you going drop** me I want my money back and I want to be **reimbused** for my time.

I initiated a conference call with the student, the chair of my department, and me, at which time the student was informed that being dropped from the course was necessary, as she had failed to meet the course requirements and would fail regardless of any future effort. (The poor grammar, spelling, punctuation, and overall negative attitude were also evident in all of her submitted assignments.)

lounge is determined by the faculty member. Students may be given free reign in communicating with one another in the student lounge for the duration of the course, or there may be specific guidelines to follow. Make certain you understand the rules for the student lounge. Faculty members also vary in their approach to the student lounge. While some may check in to the lounge occasionally in order to confirm the appropriateness of what is being discussed, others may stay out entirely once the initial introductions have been completed. If faculty do not have this specifically addressed for your course, make sure to ask. The student lounge also serves as a great place to share your thoughts with your peers and to bounce creative ideas off of one another. The possibilities of new friendships exist, but be sure to err on the side of caution so that you do not make anyone uncomfortable with your advances.

Student Lounge Use

The student lounge is a great place to share ideas or get ideas from others, just as long as it is done in a nonthreatening, collegial environment. Avoid using the student lounge as your personal forum for expressing personal beliefs or thoughts about topics such as religion, politics, or philosophy, which may cause conflict or lead to tense encounters. You may also find new opportunities by chatting with peers, or you may develop a few great friendships or long-lasting relationships on a professional level. Chat carefully, though, and if any encounter makes you feel uncomfortable, step away immediately and report it to the appropriate faculty member.

> **Student Lounge**
>
> Throughout my master's program in nursing, the faculty would clearly list the required elements for introducing ourselves to our peers in the student lounge. As time progressed, and many of us were in the same class semester after semester, faculty members changed what was required for our initial posting. Initially, we had to post our specialty area, years in nursing, physical location, and at least three facts about our life outside of school. By the end of the program, faculty required students to identify personal learning goals for the course, along with a few other unusual items. I developed several close friendships with those peers whom I met in the student lounge. Our similarities in work specialties or other common denominators bonded us together. I still maintain some of those friendships now and have used many of those contacts to further my exposure to different practices. Those who were not interested in discussing personal matters, but only class items, made their requests clear. Everyone then honored those requests.

Preventing Plagiarism

Plagiarism is a form of cheating tantamount to intellectual property theft (Moore, 2000). The academic world has strict rules concerning plagiarism, simply because it does exist and has serious consequences. Thankfully, however, it is usually the students who worry the most about plagiarism that make sure credit is given where due.

General Guidelines and Common Sense

The general rule of thumb in preventing accusations of plagiarism is simple. Always give credit where it is due. Faculty teaching in their areas of expertise will easily spot plagiarism from familiar sources. Numerous Internet resources exist for verifying whether information has been copied inappropriately and without credit. Changing just a couple of words in a sentence does not relieve you from your duty to acknowledge the source. Cite all of your references, quotes, and sources. Respect and follow all copyright agreements. Very few items in print, including those items found on the Internet, are without copyright, so be careful. Don't let plagiarism keep you from being successful in your coursework.

Consequences of Plagiarism

For almost all universities, plagiarism has serious consequences. At a minimum, students typically receive a zero grade for the assignment on which the plagiarism occurred. Other consequences may include the student failing the course or receiving an incomplete grade, necessitating the student having to repeat the course the following semester. Other academic institutions may have even more serious consequences for proof of plagiarism, such as the student's expulsion from the university overall. This is no different in the online setting of academia. The standard of ethics is not lowered just because you are participating in an online educational environment.

Shared Papers

Sharing papers is the concept of exchanging assignments among students for the express purpose of copying them and submitting that copied work for a grade. Having someone else complete your assignment and then presenting it as your own to a faculty member also constitutes plagiarism. There are numerous Web sites and software packages available to faculty members that can be used to check if students are plagiarizing other student papers or printed formats. Especially if you are using a paper previously submitted to your school, faculty members will have cause to ask around if the newly submitted assignment is of a different caliber than what you have been submitting throughout the course.

Web Sites

Turnitin.com, SafeAssign, and other companies have databases for faculty to compare submitted homework for instances of plagiarism. However, faculty members have found bugs in these programs, and they are by no means foolproof. Faculty members will always confirm a suspicion of plagiarism prior to making any kind of formal accusation. In addition to using these Web sites, faculty members may choose to vary assignments for the same course each time it is offered. It is then obvious if a student has plagiarized from another student, as his or her answers are inappropriate for the assignment. Online computer programs are also available for download to fight plagiarism. These programs allow faculty to ensure that students are unable to access another Web site or folder on their computer while answering exam questions in the online setting.

Conclusion

Communicating effectively in the online environment can be done. Assure that you adhere to proper netiquette, avoid common pitfalls, and admit when you have done something wrong, working quickly to remedy the situation. Successful communication via email can be accomplished with spelling and grammar checks, read and delivery receipts, and double checking who you are sending an email to prior to clicking the Send button. Don't get overwhelmed, but take the time to check what you have done before you post or send. By using these described methods, you will be off to a great start in communicating by computer.

Checklist for Successful Online Communication

_______ Observe the rules of netiquette.

- _______ Avoid the use of emoticons and all caps.
- _______ Select read and delivery receipts for sending an email.
- _______ Use an appropriate font size and color.

_______ Post comments that meet the guidelines or the assignment requirements.

_______ Provide proper references for all sources to avoid plagiarism.

_______ Perform spelling/grammar checks and make the recommended changes.

_______ Review the assignment in its entirety for correctness.

_______ Make sure the email or post has an appropriate subject/title.

_______ Use appropriate tone with positive statements.

_______ Verify that the email message is addressed to the correct person.

_______ Clear the list of previously sent to email addresses when forwarding an email.

_______ Convey respect by proper use of titles.

References

Aranda, J. F. (2007, Fall). Netiquette and online communication [Electronic version]. *Journal of Instruction Delivery Systems, 21*(4), 11–14.

Federal Trade Commission. (2008). *Spam.* Retrieved January 6, 2008, from http://www.ftc.gov/spam

Hoffman, P. (1999, October). *Usability interface. Accommodating color blindness.* Retrieved April 24, 2009, from http://www.stcsig.org/usability/newsletter/9910-color-blindness.html

Moore, P. (2000). *What is plagiarism?* Retrieved September 9, 2009, from http://www.mantex.co.uk/samples/plgrsm.htm

Schrauf, R. (2005). *Study: Negative words dominate language.* Retrieved January 29, 2009, from http://abcnews.go.com/Technology/DyeHard/Story?id=460987&page=1

Shay, V. (2008). *Netiquette.* Retrieved October 2, 2008, from http://www.albion.com/netiquette

The Virginia Adult Learning Resource Center. (2007). *How to be a good online learner.* Retrieved October 1, 2008, from http://www.valrc.org/tutorials/fset/communication2.htm

Chapter 10

Managing Group Assignments in the Online Learning Environment

Patricia Lisk and Katherine Quartuccio

As challenging as group work can be for students, interaction with classmates in group settings can prepare you for the complex social interactions that you will face in your professional careers. Students relate that they feel positive about the growth and the changes that occur as they work in groups. Students also report that working in groups has helped them to learn the value of teamwork and the value of their peers even in the midst of conflict. According to Dunaway (2005), students appreciate the addition of group work to their class as they believe that this learning strategy enhances their knowledge acquisition.

This chapter provides online students with information that will elucidate the historical perspective of group assignments, illuminate the online group project environment, and comment on identifiers and strategies for effective communication, management of assignments, and conflict resolution when working in groups.

Historical Perspective of Group Assignments

Group or team assignments have been used successfully in business and educational settings for more than 25 years (Michaelson, Knight, & Fink, 2002). In the educational setting, the group assignment affords the student the opportunity to become more familiar with the many aspects of group processes and group dynamics. Additionally, because it is both cooperative and interactive, group assignments allow students to confront and internalize new realities instead of just passively receiving concepts and information. Working in groups also offers to the student learning resources that are beyond their individual repertoires (Wilson, Anderson, Peluso, Priest, & Speer, 2009). Over the years, this teaching strategy has been purported to enhance critical thinking, promote active learning, and encourage group collaboration and problem solving. It has also been thought to emulate some of the complex social interactions that occur within the business and healthcare environments, thus preparing students for their careers and their professional experiences following graduation (Feingold et al., 2008).

Online Group Assignments

While many students prefer to work individually to complete course assignments, group projects provide environments for individuals to develop effective team skills that carry into the work organization. The brilliant Thomas Edison worked with a team of twenty-one. When questioned why he worked with so many people, he stated "If I could solve all the problems myself, I would" (Heartquotes Center, 2009). Group assignments lead to the development of smaller learning communities within the bigger online classroom. As these smaller learning communities work together to achieve a goal, they can serve as forum for growth of the individual members and growth of the group (see Figure 10-1).

Getting Started

While many group members are designated by faculty members in an ad hoc manner, discovering group member strengths and weaknesses should be an immediate focus for the development of group work. Each team member needs to take an honest look at the skills in which they feel they are most competent in performing and those in which they feel need further development. Some of the skills include writing, formatting, researching, communicating, and meeting deadlines. After an honest personal assessment is made, this information should be shared with the group so project parts can be assigned. This information exchange among the team members promotes cohesion within the group and, if managed carefully, provides the means for individual skill improvement (see Box 10-2).

Collaboration

Collaboration is important because it fosters a learning environment based on trust and openness. Collaboration for the completion of online group assignments can be accomplished with electronic means such as an electronic blackboard or email or through sched-

FIGURE 10-1 The Effect of Group Learning Assignments

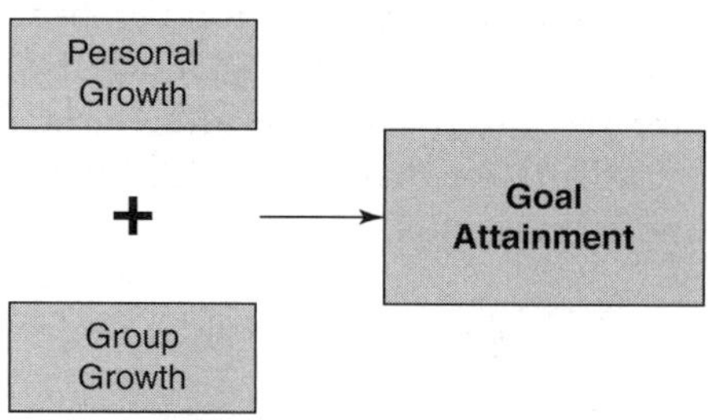

uled phone meetings. Designated means of communication for collaboration must be selected prior to project development (see Box 10-1). Each method for collaboration depends upon group member availability or available technology. According to Katzenbach and Smith (as cited in Parker, 2003), "every virtual team should develop their own 'netiquette' by discussing how they expect to apply technology to help complete their task and, when possible, agree on the selection of the [method] that the team will employ" (p. 188).

Expectations

Online learning groups should delineate role expectations for each assignment at the beginning of the group assignment in order to avoid role ambiguity. Expectations include deadlines, level of participation, and quality of submitted work (see Figure 10-2). Articulating

Box 10-1 Suggestions for Online Collaboration

- ***Establish communication methods***. This should be initiated when groups are assigned or selected. For example, each group member should check in to the online forum once per day or once per week.
- ***Create an assignment agreement***. Agreements should address project part deadlines, project expectations such as grammar and format, and conflict management strategies.
- ***Establish communication rules***. If phone conversations are used, rules should be established that will address how information will be shared with the entire group.
- ***Establish deadlines***. Provide time for project revisions or alterations in the project plan.
- ***Establish communication rules***.
    - Accept all opinions and decisions.
    - Do not force your opinion.
    - Agree to *respectfully* disagree.

FIGURE 10-2 Expectations of Group Members

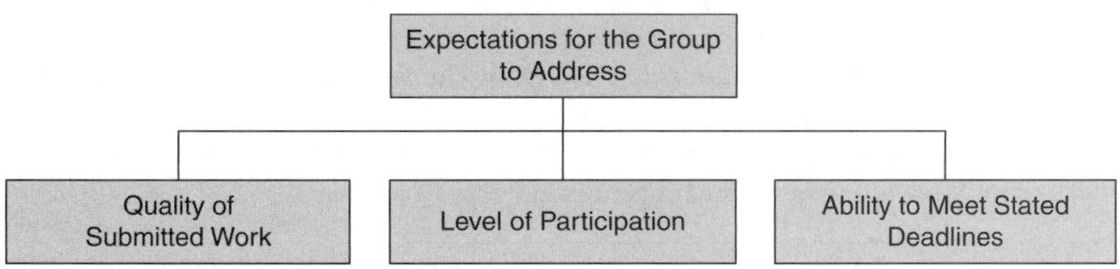

needed project skills, individual learning needs, and desired learning minimizes unrealistic or undeclared expectations.

Group Skills Development

Necessary skills for the development of group cohesion in an online environment include leadership skills, understanding of group dynamics, knowledge of needed strategies for group project completion, respect for group members, group member commitment, and the desire to complete a quality group project (Leggat, 2007). In addition to these critical skills for group assignment completion, individual skills needed include the ability to initiate projects, influence other group members, analyze project components, provide constructive feedback, and manage time effectively. Group members present with some,

Box 10-2 Case Study, Part 1

Jenny has been assigned to an online group for the completion of a health education pamphlet for diabetes education. Her team consists of three other online classmates. The pamphlet is due 2 weeks after the groups have been assigned. Previously, Jenny was part of an online group that completed a care map for congestive heart failure. Unfortunately, the group did not begin the assignment until 3 days before the due date, and Jenny needed to complete sections of the care map that were missing or inadequate. The situation was frustrating for Jenny. How should Jenny approach this group assignment?

Questions to Consider:

- What skills are necessary for completing a health education pamphlet for diabetes (i.e., research, writing, formatting, organizing)?
- What is the availability of the team members?
- When should project parts be submitted?
- Who should complete the final edit of the pamphlet?
- Who should lead the project?

Suggestion

Since Jenny recognizes the need for project initiation she may want to express her desire to begin the project in the first week, stating that this will provide time for the group to evaluate the quality of the work prior to submission. Jenny may choose to take the role of leader or she may solicit another team member's leadership.

Jenny's skill in initiating group work for assignments may provide other group members with an example of expedient work completion and goal attainment.

none, or (rarely) all of these skills. According to Leggat (2007), "The ability to perform an activity, a skill, can be the result of natural talent or acquired through education or training" (p. 5).

Group Communication

According to De Janasz, Dowd, and Schneider (2002), characteristics of highly effective teams include regular communication that keeps members informed of changes, expectations, and progress. Effective communication provides information that is clearly understood by group members, information for member reflections, and direction that leads to the group members' ability to act. Communication that does not motivate group members leads to conflict and division that is adverse to group goal attainment. Considering the overall purpose of group communication requires students contemplate content, tone, and necessity of information within the online learning environment.

One From Many

Online group assignments propose to create learning environments that promote team-learning skills that include the ability to communicate to various group/team members and create one voice that leads to improved outcomes, as demonstrated by quality project completion. In order for any group to communicate effectively, individuals must recognize the components of communication. Basic communication goes two ways: sending and receiving. Both directions of communication entail perception and interpretation on the part of the individual sending the message and the individual receiving the message.

According to Ebojo (2009), effective communication is multifaceted and is emotionally intelligent, sensitive to covert meanings, and integrates multiple communication styles. Emotional intelligence refers to the sender's and receivers' ability to handle their emotions as is fitting to the situation and their ability to manage relationships accordingly. Individuals who are emotionally intelligent are able to consider the perspective of other group members, are able to be empathetic to the situations or perspectives of group members, and are able to modify communication modes according to the situation. In face-to-face group settings, sensitivity to covert and overt tones would include body language or changes in tone of voice. In an online communication setting, effective communication considers words, context of statements, and the use of symbols such as emoticons. Ebojo (2009) considers flexibility key to effective communication that encourages group member openness and optimum participation.

Online Communication

Communication required for online group assignments necessitates patience, tolerance, focus, and contemplation. Due to the fact that online communication lacks nonverbal cues, individual responses may be interpreted as offensive or threatening. In an online environment, therefore, responses and statements should be carefully considered before hitting the Send button. According to Know Your World (2007), online communication provides an alternative method for communication requiring rules that are labeled netiquette. These netiquette rules include the need for clarity in order to unmistakably make your point; posting only statements that you would consider stating face to face; using correct grammar and abbreviations; considering font and color; and understanding that all capital letters indicate shouting. In addition to considering these netiquette rules, before sending any message, remember that once the message posts, the contents become public and can generally not be rescinded.

In order for groups to complete assignments, decisions must be made regarding goals, individual assignments, expectations, and deadlines. The group makes these decisions though productive communication. A breakdown in communication can lead to division or competition among team members that can result in a less-than-quality assignment (Porter, 2003).

Managing Group Assignments

In order to create successful assignments, designated groups must begin with a detailed assignment plan. Beginning with the selection of a leader, the team leader should develop assignment plans that include project parts, word counts, and additional expectations such as plagiarism check submissions. The project plan should be developed as soon as the group members have been assigned to their online group. The project plan should delineate member parts according to the grading criteria and grading rubric and it should include submission dates for individual parts. In addition to submission dates, the project plan should also designate one person to compile the assignment and one person to complete the first draft. This plan should be considered for group assignments such as papers or PowerPoint presentations. Incorporating assignment plans provide groups with organization and structure that promote success.

Group Stages of Development

According to De Janasz and colleagues (2002), organized groups follow a pattern of development. The steps of group development include "forming, storming, norming, performing, and adjourning" (p. 316).

Forming Stage

During the forming stage, group members discover qualities of other team members, designate parts of assignments, outline assignment objectives and work to discover the needed resources for assignment completion. During this phase of development, one group member may take the lead in managing the group assignment and outlining deadlines, establishing expectations for written projects, and providing a breakdown of the assignment.

Storming Stage

In the storming stage of group development, the group experiences "differences over factors such as direction, leadership, work style and approach, and perceptions about the expected quality and state of the end product or deliverable" (De Janasz et al., 2002, p. 315). Working with individual group members' differences requires conflict resolution that will ensure group acceptance of group leadership and group decisions that will foster group goal attainment. If this is not accomplished the group will remain in a state of nonproductive confusion.

Norming Stage

During the norming stage of group growth, members establish acceptable communication behaviors, recognize group leadership, and incorporate new methods for group assignment completion.

Performing Stage

Once the group has developed standards and expectations during the norming phase, the members enter the performing phase, in which group members focus on the goal of project completion. During the phase of performing, individual group members must focus on the group objectives and shift from personal preferences to the global perspective that leads to cooperation and acceptance.

Adjourning Stage

Upon completion of the group assignment, group members experience adjourning. Depending upon the group experience, individual members can experience frustration that the group experience has ended or they can experience relief that the group has completed the task and no longer depends upon one another for goal attainment.

The Overall Goal

Whether groups meet face to face or in the online environment, the overall goal is to create an atmosphere that is productive and positive. Effective groups demonstrate the ability to consider the opinions of others, accept leadership, center attention on the assignment, and develop successful conflict resolution methods (De Janasz et al., 2002). In order to create learning environments that are positive, group members must deliberately apply communication skills, collaboration skills, and personal responsibility for behaviors. In essence, effective groups require effective group members.

Conflict Management

No matter how carefully groups have followed these suggestions for communication and collaboration, conflict within the group is often inevitable. De Janasz and colleagues (2002) describe conflict as a situation in which groups or individuals have contradictory goals, thoughts, or feelings that lead to antagonistic communication and exchange. Often the wishes, values, and ideas of the individuals within a group are diverse, making agreement and online discussion between members difficult. At times, group members begin to feel as if consensus will never be achieved as one member or more members continue to stand in the way of problem resolution, goal attainment, and project completion.

Conflict by nature can be somewhat uncomfortable, and it may initially seem as though it is impeding progress toward group goals and objectives. The fact is, group conflict can be either bad or good. Group conflict, when handled and viewed appropriately by the group, can actually lead the group to higher levels of collaboration, creativity, and project performance. In contrast, if the conflict is approached improperly, the problem can often exacerbate and then become the demise of the group and its assigned project.

Reasons for Conflict

Let's examine some of the common reasons for conflicts within groups (see Figure 10-3). First, groups are made up of individuals who possess different talents, strengths, intellectual abilities, and personalities. Add to these factors the fact that all groups are not created equal—some groups by nature and composition are just more adversarial than others. By teasing apart some of these elements, members will be better able to understand how to approach group work and how to effectively reach collaborative performance.

Potential Source of Conflict No. 1: Goals and Objectives

Students experience conflict when members of the group have inherent differences in the goals and objectives for the group. This may at first seem odd or even impossible as the objectives for most class and group activities have been carefully laid out by the instructor. Irrespective, conflicts do arise. Conflicts arise when members are deciding who will complete the differing

FIGURE 10-3 Sources of Group Conflict

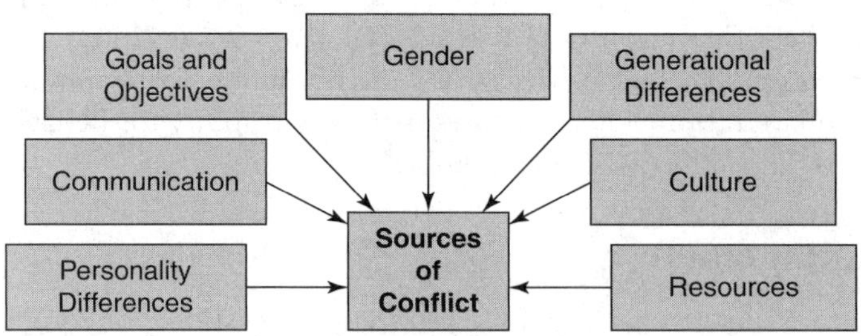

portions of the project and then how the work will be allocated and accomplished. Members may disagree about the expected quality of the final deliverable. Some members may expect a superior product, whereas other members may be content with a satisfactory product.

Potential Source of Conflict No. 2: Resources

Students often encounter conflict when discussing the resources that will be needed to complete an assignment. Frequently, students disagree about the amount of time, work, and effort that will be needed to accomplish the deliverable. Conflict may arise when select group members coast along, neglecting their group assignments, requiring other members to compensate for their lack of participation. At times, financial resources will be needed as well. As some students have limited funds, group members may disagree regarding the expenses associated with the project.

Potential Source of Conflict No. 3: Communication

As discussed earlier in this chapter, communication is one of the keys to successful group work. Communicating clearly and effectively can be challenging in a face-to-face setting. Add the dimension of online communication, which lacks nonverbal cues, and group members may inadvertently interpret constructive messages as offensive or even adversarial. In the asynchronous environment, hours or days may pass before the true intent of a well-meaning message can be clarified. During this time, negative emotions and feelings that could adversely impact the dynamics of the group may have needlessly transpired. Carefully adhering to the elements of netiquette and the principles of effective online communication outlined earlier in this text can prevent unnecessary conflict.

Potential Source of Conflict No. 4: Personality Differences

Personality differences can impact group dynamics and function as well. An obvious example of a personality conflict that may affect cohesive group function would be between a type A personality and a type B personality. The type A personality would likely be well organized and more adherent to group deadlines. The type B personality would typically be more laid back about the assignment and their portion of the project. Personality conflicts are not limited to those of type A and type B personalities; other personality conflicts will likely emerge as you are working on group assignments. It is easy to see how these opposing personalities could come into conflict when the assignment due date is rapidly approaching and stress levels are heightened.

Potential Source of Conflict No. 5: Culture, Gender, and Generation

Cultural, gender, and generational diversity may cause conflict when working in groups. Each group member brings with him or her these set factors that will affect his or her values, perceptions, and attitudes while completing group assignments. Individuals from diverse cultures have differing perspectives that need to be considered and respected when completing group assignments. Male and female dynamics and communication differences are evident within the group setting. Role taking, power assumption, and communication vary within groups where there are gender differences (Kaenzig, Hyatt, & Anderson, 2007). Generational conflict frequently occurs when group members are discussing workload and work allocation. Classically, group members falling into the baby boomer generation will value hard work and success at almost any cost, while the generations that follow will seek more balance in their lives with work assuming less importance.

Communication styles differ within the generations as well. Some generations are more flexible and tolerant; others are more rigid, while some generations have even been described as self-absorbed (Smola & Sutton, 2002). In all cases—cultural, gender, and generational—group members must recognize and appreciate the differences and diversity. When valued and embraced, these differences will add a new richness to the group collaboration and assignment completion.

Management of Conflict

Now that you are aware of some of the factors that lead to conflict, knowing how to handle the conflict will enhance your group process and group interaction. As mentioned earlier, some conflict is inevitable as the sources of conflict are apparent in almost all group interactions.

Individuals who are involved in conflict in general handle these conflicts in one of the following ways: avoidance, accommodation, competition, compromise, or collaboration (Thomas, 2002). Other individuals may include the use of conflict resolution models, such as Wisinski's A-E-I-O-U model, or a personal conflict resolution framework. No one way of handling conflict is superior to another; the best resolution often depends upon the situation surrounding the conflict. Each strategy has its own unique advantages and disadvantages and these will be discussed in detail in the following section.

Avoidance

Avoidance is the conflict resolution strategy used when individuals or groups choose not to deal with the issues or with the individuals involved in the conflict. Often when this style of conflict resolution is chosen, the issues are trivial and are not central to the work of the team. Sometimes the conflict is intentionally put aside so that the actual work of the team can be accomplished. An example of this type of conflict resolution might be intentionally to put the issue of where to have a face-to-face team social gathering temporarily on hold during an online discussion so that group members can focus on more urgent team objectives.

Avoidance Danger

One of the dangers of using the avoidance style of conflict resolution is that issues that are set to the side may worsen and become more complex as group members have agreed to avoid their discussion. Sometimes dealing with issues as they occur leads to easier resolution.

Accommodation

Accommodation is the conflict resolution style that is selected when one individual gives in to the wishes or desires of other group members. When using this method of resolution, members of the group believe that maintaining harmony and cohesiveness within the group is more important than accomplishing the objective of the group.

Accommodation Danger

One of the dangers of consistently choosing this style of conflict resolution is that if the group always chooses this method of resolution, it may sacrifice group goals for the maintenance of the group relationship. Additionally, over time, individuals who consistently submit to the wishes of the group may harbor resentment over unmet ideas and suggestions.

Competition

Competition occurs when a group member believes that his or her ideas are so important or accurate that the team member aggressively works to achieve these perspectives regardless of the cost to the group. Often the group member believes that the pursued approach is the only right one and is ready to sacrifice group relationships to see the idea adopted. When emergency or urgent group situations arise that require immediate decisions, this conflict management style is often selected.

Competition Danger

One of the clear dangers of using this method of conflict resolution is that there are clear winners and losers in the situation, hence leading to potential divisiveness within the group.

Compromise

Compromise occurs when team members are having difficulty coming to a decision. In this situation, each of the competing factions gives up a portion of its perspective for the sake of group agreement. There is no clear winner as each faction has conceded and is only partially satisfied with the decision. This conflict management style is frequently used by group members when the deadline for the project is approaching, and a compromise is the easiest and perhaps the best decision that can be reached in the remaining time.

Compromise Danger

The danger of consistently using this type of problem solving is that part of the group goal and group relationship may be consciously sacrificed to solve the issue.

Collaboration

Collaboration is the conflict management style that is selected when group members are interested in finding a solution that meets all the ideas and perspectives of individual group members. This style requires excellent online communication skills as group members must be able to express dissatisfaction in a constructive manner and then continue to work towards new and creative solutions to the problem as well as project completion.

> **Collaboration Danger**
>
> The greatest obstacle to this conflict management style is time. Each group member must allocate sufficient time and energy to reach a solution that is acceptable to all members of the group. In the online environment, this is a time consuming yet rewarding undertaking. Not all members are willing to make such a sacrifice. At times, project deadlines may be exceeded or members may default to another style of problem solving.

A-E-I-O-U Model

Wisinski's (1993) A-E-I-O-U model helps groups clearly delineate problems or conflicts and then prepares the group to suggest possible solutions. When a conflict arises, before engaging in further group discussions, each team member is encouraged to engage in and follow the steps to the model described next (see Figure 10-4).

A—*Assume the Other Group Members Mean Well* In step A, you and your group members must *assume* that all members are interested in positive group interactions and successful proj-

FIGURE 10-4 Wisinski's A-E-I-O-U Model

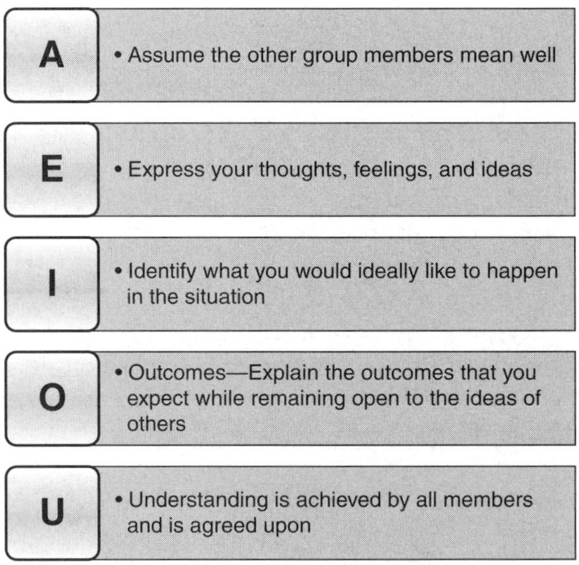

Source: Adapted from Wisinski, 1993.

ect completion. During this step, members express willingness to work with one another and a confidence that all members are concerned about the success of the group.

E—*Express Your Thoughts, Feelings, and Ideas* In step E, you and members of your group vent and *express* feelings about actions and events that have occurred within the group. When individuals express their perceptions of group problems, the group can then assess the situation or conflict with more clarity.

I—*Identify What You Would Ideally Like to Happen in the Situation* In step I, you, along with other group members, have the opportunity to *identify* what you would like to see happen in the situation. During this step, the group will be able to consider multiple ideas and solutions to the problem at hand.

O—*Explain the Outcomes That You Expect While Remaining Open to the Ideas of Others* In step O, you and your team members discuss possible *outcomes* of the conflict—both positive and negative. Group members may begin to discuss fears and concerns associated with project deadlines and project completion.

U—*Understanding Is Achieved by All Members and Is Agreed Upon* In the final step, U, you and your fellow group members discuss all available options and move to an agreement on one of the possible solutions. Each team member should *understand* and commit to the agreed-upon solution to the conflict at this time (Wisinski, 1993).

Conflict Resolution Processes

After the problem has been explored and you and your group members are fully acquainted with the nature of the conflict, the resolution processes of consensus, voting, mediation, and arbitration are additional strategies to help you resolve the conflict (see Figure 10-5).

FIGURE 10-5 Conflict Resolution Processes

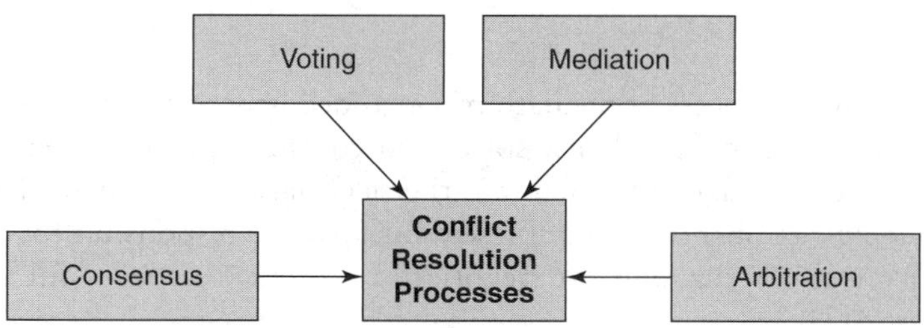

Consensus

The conflict resolution process of consensus is used when the group is unable to come to a unanimous decision. According to Porter (2004), consensus exists when all members of the group are able to support a group-chosen decision and put aside any lingering doubts, questions, and reservations about the decision. Consensus requires that all members thrash out their views on issues that are central to the group's conflict and then bargain with one another to settle differences and reach solutions. Most teams use this informal process to solve conflicts. In an online environment, group members would need to indicate consensus at some point. A designated member could check for consensus among group members by periodically asking the question, "Could all members of the group support this chosen decision?" If all members concur, a consensus has been reached, and team members can move forward to the next element of their assignment.

If groups are having difficulty generating solutions to conflict, brainstorming is a method that can be used to formulate potential solutions. When groups brainstorm, as many ideas as possible are identified without actually considering the feasibility of any of the solutions. In a face-to-face environment, students orally exchange thoughts and ideas. In the online environment, students contribute and exchange ideas in written form for group review and evaluation. After all members have contributed possible solutions, group members evaluate the solutions for one that is creative yet feasible and is in concurrence with the objectives of the assignment.

Voting

Sometimes groups resolve conflict by allowing members to cast a vote on the issue being considered. In this case, a simple majority is usually considered sufficient to carry the decision. When using voting as a conflict resolution process, the group must be cognizant of the fact that when a group reaches a decision through voting there will be definite winners and losers. Unless an online survey tool is used in the online environment, there will be no anonymity in the voting process. All members will know who voted for and who voted against a certain aspect of the project. As noted earlier in this chapter, when there are definite losers and winners within a group, this division can lead to erosion of group morale through conscious or subconscious actions of the members (Porter, 2004).

Mediation

The conflict resolution process of mediation is a guided negotiation process. When team members are not able to independently solve their conflicts, members may ask a faculty member or outside third party to facilitate the negotiation or to help them solve the conflict. The faculty member or the nonbiased third party is responsible for coaching and guiding group members through the negotiation process to successful resolution of conflict (Porter, 2003).

Arbitration

The conflict resolution process of arbitration is rarely used in academic group negotiation. This type of resolution process is used when a group's conflict is at an impasse and group members are unwilling to negotiate or reach an agreement. With arbitration, an arbitrator will consider all group options selected. The arbitrator may select one of the options or in some cases may develop an innovative solution that has not even been considered by the group. In either case, all team members must abide by the decision of the arbitrator. With this type of conflict resolution, again, there are definite winners and losers, which may lead to team division and a decline in group morale (Porter, 2003).

Cohesion

As you probably know if you have ever interacted or worked within a group, conflict can be stressful and absorbs much of the time that might be used for project completion. Groups that can effectively solve their conflicts and work together to achieve group goals in a cohesive fashion are those that will be most successful. According to Engleberg, Wynn, and Schuttler (2003), cohesion is the mutual attraction that pulls group members together and augments group performance. Because cohesive groups are more satisfied, feel more committed, and use more creative and productive approaches when achieving goals, you may want to undertake strategies in your group to enhance its cohesion. Several strategies have been suggested to enhance group cohesion, enhance group performance, and prevent irresolvable conflict (Bormann & Bormann, 1996). These are as follows:

- *Establish an identity*—Start by referring to your group and group members using terms such as *we* or *our*. This type of language helps to encourage interconnectedness among group members.
- *Emphasize group work*—Each member needs to take responsibility for contributing regularly to the function of the group. Group members need to make comments and statements emphasizing the importance of each member's role, as it relates to the contribution to the group. In an online environment, some members may believe that it is easy to step away from regular posting and scheduled input. Instead of recognizing a single individual's contributions, recognize how the contributions of all members influence progress towards group goals.
- *Appreciate and acknowledge contributions*—Often, group members become so involved in their own contributions to the group that they neglect to recognize and praise others' contributions. While providing constructive criticism is necessary for a quality group project, consciously taking time to praise and recognize the efforts of group members is an important balance.
- *Respect members of the group*—If you and your group regularly require members to complete their part of the project without regard for their individual needs and

concerns, little cohesion will develop within the group. Most members will have an occasion where turning in an assignment may become challenging because of a life-altering event. Treating members with respect and showing concern during these times helps to create more cohesion within the group. Similarly, in consideration for all group members, individuals should routinely post work and assigned activities in a timely fashion, thereby demonstrating respect for the needs of other members within the group who may be compiling and placing the final touches on the group assignment.

Although cohesion is a desirable outcome for groups, a certain amount of conflict is desirable as well. Groups that are highly cohesive are at risk of developing groupthink. Groupthink is a condition characterized by the corrosion of the effectiveness of the group when it succumbs to internal pressure from members to conform (Engleberg et al., 2003). To avoid groupthink, members need to remember that the expression of group differences is just as important as achieving group consensus. Encourage group members to offer opposing views. Perhaps it could be the assignment of one of the members to simply ask questions and look at the negative aspect of each suggestion. In short, this individual would be assigned to create conflict. Without some conflict, creativity and unique approaches are often overlooked.

Case Study

Let's examine again our case study (see Box 10-3) where Jenny and her classmates have been assigned a care mapping project. This time, let's focus on some of the inherent differences within the group. Let's focus on their conflict and explore ways that this could be resolved by the group. Test your conflict management skills by reviewing the following case study. How would you handle this situation?

Box 10-3 Case Study, Part 2

Jenny has been assigned to an online group for the completion of a health education pamphlet for diabetes education. Jenny is a 41-year-old Caucasian mother of a troubled teen. Jenny is currently in a difficult and at times abusive marriage. Jenny reads through the introductory activities for the class paying close attention to the qualities and characteristics of the members of her group. She finds that her team consists of three other online classmates whom she has never encountered in the face-to-face environment. One of the teammates is Marcus, an African American male, aged 31, and a father of three children, who is returning to school following a long history of employment as a mechanic in the airline industry. The third member of the group is a single, 25-year-old female, Lingh, an Asian student who has recently come to the United States with English as her second language. The last member of the group is a 19-year-old female, Brittany, who has five roommates and is carrying a course load of 18 credits this semester.

The pamphlet is due 2 weeks after the groups have been assigned.

One week after the project assignment, the group has run into an issue. Brittany has consistently turned her work in late and is now disagreeing with most of the suggestions offered by other members of the group. Jenny is becoming impatient with Brittany's apparent lack of commitment to the group and her deterrence of group progress through her unending "what about" questions. Marcus and Lingh are concerned that if the disagreements continue, their project will remain incomplete. Lingh does not want to sacrifice her GPA and is willing at this point to take on the entire project and complete it herself without the assistance of her group.

Questions to Consider:

- What are some of the talents, strengths, and abilities of this group?
- In what ways does this group demonstrate diversity?
- How will this diversity affect group process and conflict resolution?
- Should the group allow Lingh to complete the project? Why or why not?
- How would you suggest that the group conflict be resolved?

Suggestion

The group of students has demonstrated academic success and most of them have work and life experiences that will produce a rich and creative project. The students demonstrate gender, generational, cultural, and personality diversity. Because of the diversity, clear and frequent communication will be required for project completion. As Brittany has not been prompt in turning in her assignments, group members should explore with her the reasons for her tardiness, and when it is appropriate, be supportive of her personal needs to foster cohesion within the group. At the same time, group members need to express to Brittany that her tardiness is impeding the performance of the entire group and that the expectation is that her work needs to be completed in a timely fashion. Allowing Lingh to complete the project independently may be the easiest solution to this problem but the group project would be deprived of the creative ideas that would emerge if all members collaborated effectively. The group conflict would best be solved through brainstorming and consensus. If this issue were put to a vote, with the short amount of time left for project completion, group members would likely vote to allow Lingh to complete the project independently. Group members, however, need to consider the consequences of voting. Members should also consider Lingh's feelings and how these actions will affect future group interactions in this class.

Conclusion

The integration of group assignments into the online learning environment presents a plethora of challenges for online students. However, the attitude and manner of approaching group assignments can result not only in the development of communication and interpersonal skills necessary in today's working environment, but also contribute to the personal and intellectual growth of each individual student. It cannot be overemphasized that communication and problem-solving skills go hand in hand with successful participation and positive outcomes when engaging in group assignments. Additionally, students must bear in mind the importance that gender differences, social issues, age characteristics, and personal dynamics impact the overall ability of groups to function successfully.

Strategies for approaching group assignments in an online venue and for managing your group have been presented. The importance of clear and timely online communication has been highlighted along with some rules of netiquette and conflict resolution. Utilizing the suggested strategies in this chapter can assist in the completion of school-assigned projects as well as work projects that you may encounter in your profession.

Checklist for Managing Group Assignments

______ Determine who has been assigned to your group.

______ Discover group member strengths and weaknesses.

______ Designate a group leader.

- ______ Develop assignment plans.
- ______ Designate one person to obtain the project parts from each member.
- ______ Designate one person to complete the draft after all parts are received.

______ Establish means of communication for collaboration.

______ Delineate role expectations of each individual and of the group as a whole.

______ Create an atmosphere that is productive and positive.

- ______ Understand potential sources of conflict.
- ______ Implement strategies to handle these conflicts.

References

Bormann, E., & Bormann, N. (1996). *Effective small group communication* (6th ed., pp. 137–139). Edina, MN: Burgess Publishing.

De Janasz, S. C., Dowd, K. O., & Schneider, B. Z. (2002). *Interpersonal skills in organizations* (pp. 371-393, 241–259). New York: McGraw-Hill.

Dunaway, G. (2005). Adaptation of team learning to an introductory graduate pharmacology course. *Teaching and Learning in Medicine, 17*(1), 56–62.

Ebojo, M. (2009). Guide to skillful communication. *Pharmaceutical Executive, 9*(4), 16–18. Retrieved June 19, 2009, from EBSCO host database.

Engleberg, I., Wynn, D., & Schuttler, R. (2003). *Working in groups: Communication principles and strategies* (3rd ed., pp. 146–170). Boston: Houghton Mifflin.

Feingold, C. E., Cobb, M. D., Givens, R. H., Arnold, J., Joslin, S., & Keller, J. L. (2008). Student perceptions of team learning in nursing education. *Journal of Nursing Education, 47,* 214–222.

Heartquotes Center. (2009). *Teamwork quotes and proverbs.* Retrieved June 18, 2009, from http://www.heartquotes.net/teamwork-quotes.html

Kaenzig, R., Hyatt, E., & Anderson, S. (2007). Gender differences in college of business educational experiences. *Journal of Education for Business, 83*(2), 95–100.

Know Your World. (2007, November 2). Quit shouting and other Internet guidelines. *Know Your World Extra.* Retrieved June 19, 2009, from EBSCO host database.

Leggat, S. (2007). Effective healthcare teams require effective team members: Defining teamwork competencies. *BMC Health Services Research, 7*(17), 1–10. Retrieved June 18, 2009, from EBSCO host database.

Michaelson, L. K., Knight, A. B., & Fink, L. D. (Eds.). (2002). *Team based learning: A transformative approach use of small groups.* Westport, CT: Praeger.

Porter, S. (2003). *Managing conflict in learning teams* (pp. 1–9). Phoenix, AZ: University of Phoenix.

Porter, S. (2004). *Team decision-making* (pp. 1–13). Phoenix, AZ: University of Phoenix. Retrieved June 19, 2009, from http://www.apollolibrary.com/LTT/download/TeamDecisionMaking.pdf

Smola, M., & Sutton, C. (2002). Generational differences: Revisiting generational work values for the new millennium. *Journal of Organizational Behavior, 23*(special issue), 263–382.

Thomas, K. W. (2002). *Introduction to conflict management: Improving performance using TKI.* Palo Alto, CA: CCP, Inc.

Wilson, B., Anderson, J., Peluso, C., Priest, J., & Speer, T. (2009). Student satisfaction and team development outcomes with preassigned learning communities. *Journal of Professional Nursing, 25*(1), 15–22. Retrieved June 13, 2009, from ScienceDirect database.

Wisinski, J. (1993). *Resolving conflicts on the job.* New York: American Management Association.

Chapter 11

Enriching Your Online Experience with Collegiality

Susan Sonnier

The online classroom experience is filled with many opportunities for personal and professional growth. However, the general opinion of online learners and faculty members tends to align with that of many researchers and educational experts, in that they describe a certain element of social isolation present in the online learning environment (Aragon, 2003; Misanchuk & Anderson, 2001). This issue can pose a unique challenge for the online learning population.

Would an online peer group enhance the learning experience? Would it diminish the loneliness of the online classroom? Are online relationships and social interactions a way to address the issue of social isolation? If so, how do we form social groups or learning communities in the face of those obstacles presented by the online environment? Theoretical and practical constructs that answer these questions suggest that online collegiality and social relationships *can* make the online learning experience richer and more meaningful.

These relationships will be illustrated in this chapter in order to demonstrate the benefits of online camaraderie and collegiality. The goal of sharing these tips and real-life scenarios is to help you to understand the value of social relationships during your online learning experiences. There is a real and distinct possibility that these social interactions will help to sustain you throughout your curriculum of study.

Proliferation and Popularity of Online Learning Experiences

There is little room to dispute the proliferation and popularity of online learning experiences over the past 25 years. The Sloan Consortium's annual report on the status of online learning in the United States demonstrates clear upward trends in the number of students enrolled in online learning programs. Allen and Seaman (2008) report that "over 3.9 million students were taking at least one online course, a 12% increase over the number reported the previous year" (p. 1). Several reasons for the increased popularity and enrollment were due to higher gas prices, rising unemployment, and the need for job retraining or new skill acquisition. Colleges and universities are aware of these growing student needs and consider the availability of online courses and curriculum necessary to long-term success (Allen & Seaman).

Sociability in the Classroom: Important or Not?

It is easy to see that the online learning environment is becoming an increasingly sought-after experience for both seasoned and first-time college students. However, it can be difficult for many to be involved in a course when all you face is a flat screen with little or no contact with your instructor or classmates. Although one may argue the importance of sociability, there are definite personal and professional advantages of having a social group of colleagues who align to help you to achieve your goals in the online classroom. Some authors have termed this social interactivity *cybersolace,* or the emotional support one can receive in an electronic environment (Beder, 2005). In the next section, these benefits will be explained in better detail to help you see how social interactions can enhance your online experience.

Benefits of Social Interactions Online

Online classrooms are scattered over virtually endless locations. Distance learners may be in clustered population centers such as the upper portion of New York, where students are participating in a new online nursing bachelor's degree program (State University of New York–Delhi, 2008), or the learners can be dispersed all over the globe at national and international locations. Regardless of the milieu of the classroom participants, students can be at risk for feelings of learner isolation that is indigenous to the online learning environment (Aragon, 2003; Misanchuk & Anderson, 2001). Although these feelings of isolation are not unique or rare, they can be minimized by participating in social interactions with faculty and fellow students. There are numerous benefits of social interaction that will be explored to demonstrate the worth of these relationships in your online studies.

Connectivity

Connectivity is usually defined in the mechanical sense as the Internet connection between your computer and the host college. In this discussion of the benefits of social interactions in online environments, we will entertain another meaning of connectivity—that is, people connecting with people in the online classroom. Teaching and learning are based on social interactions between students and between faculty and students. A degree of social presence must be displayed and engaged in for the learning environment to be successful. How is that accomplished when the professor is in Springfield, Illinois, and the student is in Houston, Texas? Social presence theory suggests that participants enter varying degrees of interpersonal relationships in the mediums or mechanisms of the online learning environment. Each person must connect and share with others in order to bring about communities of learning. Faculty members can serve as role models for this connectivity. Students can then engage in these social interactions to help a program of study be a more tolerable or even pleasurable experience (Aragon, 2003).

Warm Fuzzies

There is often a degree of fear or a sense of foreboding when a person enters a new and unfamiliar environment. Online learning environments are no less intimidating for many students, especially when beginning an online program of study or entering a new online classroom. Interacting with classmates is a sure way to forge friendships with new and exciting people from all over the world and to build networks of partners with whom to study and work on projects in the classroom, and perhaps with whom to work on projects even after graduation. There are innumerable benefits that may arise from the sharing of experiences in these cyber environments, and there is much to be gained by seeking out these relationships as you begin and progress through your studies. So start feeling those warm fuzzies, and consider meeting a few classmates while you are in the online classroom!

Removing Face-to-Face Barriers to Learning

Reasons for students entering the online learning environment are as diverse as the students themselves. When asked what made the online learning environment an attractive and beneficial option to pursue a graduate degree, one student wrote the following:

> What surprised me the most about an online program was how close you could get to a person without ever having to meet them face to face. I think you could remove the distractions of sex, ethnicity, and socioeconomic status . . . all the things that could make us judge one another, and simply meet the person where they are at the time. It was very freeing to get to know someone for their "brain" first. You get to know each other and over time, you develop that lasting, deep relationship, something I rarely did in my on ground college. I truly feel these online friends I have made within the Walden walls will be lifelong friends. (J. Fomenko, personal communication, September 3, 2007)

Removing communication distracters can lead to dialogues that are more meaningful, experiences that are shared without reservation, and perceptions and opinions that are expressed more openly in the classroom. This can assist in the development of kinships and affiliations with others that will bring about a richer learning experience (Douglass, 2007; Ivankova & Stick, 2005).

Getting More Out of Your Coursework with Classmates

A distinct advantage of participating in social interactions in an online class is the benefit of constructing new knowledge with your colleagues in the classroom. The learning theory of social constructivism postulates that when learners integrate new knowledge and share personal experiences together, they can construct and formulate new knowledge that is meaningful to them (Legg, Adelman, Mueller, & Levitt, 2009). The online learning environment can be ideal for this new knowledge building.

When you have diverse colleagues with whom you feel a degree of comfort, you will elaborate upon, debate, question, define, and propose solutions to the classroom topics you will encounter in a course (Kreijns, Kirshner, Jochems, & Van Buuren, 2004). The feedback you receive from your colleagues can enrich your mastery of the subjects explored in the classroom. Learning in this manner becomes much more learner-centered, as opposed to the traditional professor-led lectures. These social interactions can lead you to a more profound and rewarding understanding of your chosen course of study (Holly, Legg, Mueller, & Adelman, 2008; Legg, Adelman, Mueller, & Levitt, 2009).

Several scholars have studied the correlation between student retention rates and the formation of online social groups in college degree programs. These scholars found two main factors to which the student's ability to remain in his or her course of study can be attributed: persistence, in which students are likely to bond over their course of study (Ivankova & Stick, 2005), and mutuality, in which learners invest in each other's ideas and thoughts as well as share ideas and solutions (Misanchuk & Anderson, 2001).

Personal Growth Through Mentoring Relationships

Mentoring is the process by which an experienced individual supports, guides, facilitates, or leads a less experienced protégé through an occurrence or course of study. Mentoring relationships can develop in any and all fields of study. A mentor can be a faculty member, a graduate student, a student who is a class ahead, or just someone who has more development in the chosen field. You may not think a mentoring-styled relationship would be possible in an electronic learning environment, but they are surprisingly prevalent (Buchanan, Myers, & Hardin, 2005; Burgess, 2007; Thomas, 2006).

Entering into a mentoring relationship can help to initially dispel some of the technical fears a student may feel as he or she begins the coursework. Burgess (2007) shares that instructors, academic advisors, or teachers' assistants are likely to be your first mentoring associates in the online platform. They often have a link to communicate your concerns and to help guide you through the initial technical maze of an online course. Online instructors or professors are trained to be sensitive to student needs and can facilitate your acclimation to the e-classroom (Burgess, 2007).

Mentoring assistance may be available to you as an offered benefit of your college or university. In this situation, a mentor volunteer has generally been assessed and trained to help you navigate difficult subject matter or to simply offer emotional support to you through a difficult period or set of assignments that may seem incomprehensible or difficult to accomplish. These types of interactions can be invaluable to you as you progress and find success in your online studies (Buchanan, Myers, & Hardin, 2005; Thomas, 2006). These mentoring individuals want you to share your successes as well. Completing your coursework and basking in that accomplishment can lead you to be the next mentor in your chosen field when a mentee is in need (Miller, Devaney, Kelley, & Kuehn, 2008).

Building Lasting Relationships for the Future

Yet another benefit of participating in classroom social interactions is the likelihood of developing lasting relationships with colleagues in your profession, or with those who are pursuing the same degree. These relationships can persist beyond graduation and can help you to navigate your new career, sustain you through personal trials, or simply be a source of enjoyment and friendship.

There are many advantages to forming some sort of social relationship while in an online classroom or learning environment. Social relationships help you to feel connected, validated, encouraged, and supported by your peers, instructors, and advisors as you progress through the required courses to complete your degree. There is no need for feelings of loneliness or isolation. You can meet many interesting and diverse types of people who can share their experiences and help you to build new meaning and acquire new knowledge. Creating and nurturing these social relationships can leave a lasting impression upon you and others. The sidebar entitled "The Master Chicks" at the end of this chapter paints a vivid example of the type of relationships that were formed and exist to this day with a group of master's degree nursing students. Hopefully, you will brave this opportunity and succeed in your endeavors.

PhinisheD

PhinisheD is an online, nonthreatening, and supportive Web site for those students working on their PhD dissertations and master's theses. Its administrator is Dr. Thomas Jankowski, a researcher and administrator at Wayne State University in Detroit, Michigan. The initial idea was born on a discussion board by Web developer Amy Bellinger. Her idea is based on a well-accepted tenet in advanced learning communities promoting assistance and support for weary graduate and postgraduate learners in their pursuit and preparation of their thesis or dissertation.

Their goal is to "promote camaraderie fellowship, and a safe outlet for venting and commiseration. PhinisheD is an antidote to other discussion forums devoted to life in academia which seem to be a little colder, a little harder, and a lot less friendly to budding scholars harboring doubts, fears, and insecurities about their lives and their work" (Phinished.org, 2008). PhinisheD is a site where a learner can meet struggling scholars and share the experiences and frustrations that come with advanced studies. The site is devoted to sharing the possibilities of online camaraderie and collegiality. You can visit the site at http://www.phinished.org.

An Alphabetic Approach to Developing Social Relationships in Online Environments

Perhaps the development of friends and colleagues sounds like a worthy pursuit. There are clear benefits to this notion of online collegiality, but a learner is likely to have many questions about it, such as: How do I go about forming these relationships? Where do I go to find these social havens for my weary mind and soul? Does the online institution have any designated student social places I can go to online? This section will help you take the steps to finding and accessing these adjuncts that can help you develop and pursue social groups in an online learning forum.

At this juncture, a simple disclaimer may be necessary to include in our discussion. There will be some students or participants who do not and will not feel comfortable interacting with others, or feel as if there is no need to form a social peer group in an online learning situation. This is a personal and private choice that each individual student will make as he or she progresses through courses. How you choose to interact with your fellow participants in a learning environment is entirely your decision. However, knowing the many and varied benefits of the online social construct, we will proceed with the how-to steps of forming social groups in the classroom for those who choose to partake in the adventure.

Step A: Acclimate and Ask Yourself

You must begin with acclimation to the online environment at the start of your online program. Getting to know the technical features of your online classroom and what your course workload will be, as well as managing the rigors of disciplining yourself to complete that coursework, will become your primary focus in the first weeks of class (Brown, 2001). Students who are beginning in online environments often have adjustments to make. This will take a considerable amount of time, so there may not be much of an opportunity to socialize or make friends.

Once you have acclimated yourself to the classroom and your schedule is working well, you will need to ask yourself how much time you want to devote to participating in the social activity in the classroom, and what types of social relationships you are interested in pursuing. The social activity and social relationships can be either formal or informal. Formal relationships are mandatory and generally revolve around the formal proceedings of the class, such as the structured lessons and weekly assignments, and include the instructor and other students. Informal relationships are voluntary and generally occur outside the realm of the classroom. The amount of time students spend socializing is often based upon individual needs and personal goals.

Dr. Diane M. Billings Comments on the Topic of Socialization in the Online Environment

Dr. Diane M. Billings, Professor Emeritus of Nursing at Indiana University, is a world renowned pioneer of distance learning in nursing. She had a personal correspondence with Sally Rudy (a simulation lab/nurse instructor at Milton S. Hershey Medical Center in Hershey, Pennsylvania) about what she felt was the importance of socializing in online environments. Dr. Billings shared the following thought with Sally: "My 'intuition' indicates support groups are essential for survival. One could hypothesize that students are more connected or feel more social presence in the course if they have these out of class experiences. So go for it!" (S. Rudy, personal communication with Dr. Diane Billings, June 21, 2007)

Step B: Borrow the Tools

Formal tools, such as the discussion threads, blackboards or whiteboards, question and answer forums, and instructor announcements, are readily available for you to begin conversations and to settle into the classroom. There is usually also a forum to share some information about yourself and to have other classmates and your instructor respond in the beginning of each class.

The informal or voluntary tools of communication with your peers may include chats, email, message boards, a student lounge, and/or a virtual café area. The student lounges and virtual cafés are generally off limits to instructors, which allows you to freely communicate with other students. This is an area where many peers can become friends and share personal experiences, frustrations, and any other information apart from the classroom milieu. While the unspoken rules of cordiality, netiquette, online manners, and self-discipline are important to follow in these informal areas, they still encourage social interactions to flourish (Tilley, Boswell, & Cannon, 2006).

Step C: Conversation and Communication

As you immerse yourself further into the social realm of the class, you will find colleagues with similar interests, opinions, motivations, and backgrounds through your communications with them (Brown, 2001). You may find there to be some degree of trust forming in sharing with one or several others. You may feel like you belong to a small group of like-minded people in the complexity and distance of the format in which you are learning. Conversation and communication are crucial here in order to foster these relationships. Be responsive and reply to the person you are attempting to befriend or who is befriending you. These relationships can heighten and enhance your learning experience greatly and can help to seed and grow learning communities as you continue in your studies.

Step D: Discover the Diversity

Diversity is a stimulating factor in any classroom. In the online learning environment, you are not able to see the age, sex, cultural, or ethnic richness in your class. You cannot imagine the gamut of differing life experiences that other students will bring to the discussions and share with you. While some of these opinions or expressions may be controversial or contrary to your own feelings or opinions, some of the best discussion threads can occur when thoughts or ideas clash. A good online tactic is to be proactive and embrace the diversity and to participate in those discussions that may be different and new to you. Many times, there can be some interesting kinships born of diversity in the online class setting.

Step E: Engage, Experience, and Experiment

Embracing the sociability that can develop in an online learning environment is undoubtedly a worthy pursuit. As you gain confidence and acceptance in the coursework with your professors and colleagues, you will find that your social circle will widen. This can be of great benefit to you in your learning experience. A widened social circle can help you in completing a group assignment or debating an issue in the classroom. More informally, a widened social circle can make you feel compelled to email a friend or two, exchange phone numbers, and talk on the phone about class issues or the commonalities you have discovered together.

Lessons in Forming Online Colleagues

A master's degree student writes a commentary for her professor at the close of a course that shares the true magnitude of communication with her peers:

> Communicating in an online group enriched the learning experience outside of the required elements of the coursework. Bonds formed to strengthen my resolve to finish the coursework when the frustrations of balancing life, work, and school were overwhelming. Without these new friends, I don't know if I would have succeeded in completing the program. (E. Pratt, personal communication, September 3, 2007)

Step F: Friendships, Families, and the Final Step

In this continuum of socialization in the online environment, you must find your comfort zone. You do not need to feel compelled to push yourself beyond your personal comfort level. You will need to determine the level at which you will be able to thrive and can continue to succeed in your studies. In addition, it is important not to leave behind the influence and support of your family and friends who were in your life before your online learning experience ever began.

These steps have been presented to help you to see the possibilities and benefits of having online relationships that can not only enhance and improve your learning experience, but also diminish the isolation a learner can perceive in a classroom of virtual strangers who may never meet face to face.

Conclusion

Online collegiality is the process by which individuals come together in a learning scenario and form personal relationships in the online environment. A dynamic learning community evolves when members treat each other and their opinions with respect, listen actively, share experience and knowledge with the others equably, and foster understanding. It is within these key community building processes that one can find collegiality and interaction with others. Through these interactions, we enhance our own learning and not only build our own knowledge base but create a common and collective base of learning that is beneficial to all.

The Master Chicks

In this sidebar, you will meet a unique group of women known as the Master Chicks. These women began the Walden University master of science in nursing degree program in 2005. They bonded together over a period of 2 years to become a formidable and lasting group of friends all over the United States. Their legacy and kinship are still spoken of in Walden University circles to this day. They are a testament to the wealth and worth of friendships that can be found and enjoyed in online learning communities.

A chapter on online collegiality would not be complete without the story of the Master Chicks. This band of 14 females came together over a period of as many months as they were enrolled in master's studies at Walden University. They shared classes together in the beginning and found some commonalities and interests that compelled them to seek each other out in the student lounge. Things that drew them together at first were living in Texas, poetry, family stories, and a professor who modeled and shared much of herself in the classroom. They had several discussions that always seemed to lead to silliness and common expressed opinions. The student lounge became a place to visit and share much about themselves. They began to share more out of the classroom when they had a difficult instructor. They banded together as the Six Chicks to demonstrate solidarity on an issue to the instructor. The issue has long been forgotten, but the endearment and kinship that developed was a lasting residual of that event.

As the first year ended, they had shared many professional and personal successes and calamities, and they were leading into the specialization coursework. Half of the Six Chicks went into a leadership/management path and the other half into the education track. The leader of the group felt compelled to garner some new friends to help her deal with the rigors of the coursework ahead. Eight more individuals joined the original group and began the same collegiality and camaraderie that had been modeled with the Six Chicks. Online introductions and initiations were in order, and the Six Chicks became the Master Chicks in a unanimous vote. They had a league of supportive and cooperative relationships that sustained and carried them to their graduation destination in 2008. Then they finally met face to face and not only shared the mountaintop experience of graduation and the attainment of their degrees, but celebrated the associations and friendships that had grown out of an online experience.

One of the Master Chicks fondly reflected and wrote this remembrance:

> We had nothing to lose, but everything to gain by participating and interacting together. Ours was a culture within a culture that developed to sooth and nurture the online traveler on a short journey. Some of us took what we needed from this time and moved on. For others, we have continued these symbiotic relationships and embraced them even after graduation. The collegiality that grew out of these basic survival needs blossomed into lifetime lessons of friendship. (K. Stanley, personal communication to Susan Sonnier, February 28, 2009)

Checklist to Identify How You Feel About Online Collegiality

Answer the questions in this checklist honestly. If you mark more yes answers than no answers, it is very likely the experience of online friends and colleagues would be of benefit as you pursue your course of study.

Yes	No	
_______	_______	Do you want to enrich your online learning experience in a positive and meaningful way?
_______	_______	Do you think you would like to engage in forming and maintaining an online learning community?
_______	_______	Do you feel the development of social interactions with others may help you enjoy the classes more? Do you feel these new colleagues would help you reach your goal of completing your courses?
_______	_______	Do you feel you could learn more through sharing your experiences and through the shared experience of others in your online class?
_______	_______	Would you benefit from a mentoring relationship in your course of study?
_______	_______	Do you feel acclimated enough to your learning environment to begin online relationships with your cohorts?
_______	_______	Have you found the social forum or location within your virtual classroom where you can socialize with others?
_______	_______	Are you willing to seek out or lead the efforts to form online learning groups or social groups in your classes?

References

Allen, E. I., & Seaman, J. (2008, November). Staying the course: Online education in the United States, 2008. *The Sloan Consortium*. Needham, MA. Retrieved January 16, 2009, from http://www.sloan-c.org/publications/survey/index.asp

Aragon, S. R. (2003, Winter). Creating social presence in online environments [Electronic version]. *New Directions for Adult Learning and Continuing Education, 100*, 57–68.

Beder, J. (2005). Cybersolace: Technology built on emotion. *Social Work, 50*(4). Retrieved August 7, 2007, from Academic Search Database.

Brown, R. E. (2001). The process of community building in distance learning classes [Electronic version]. *Journal for Asynchronous Learning Networks, 5*(2), 18–34. Retrieved February 27, 2009, from http://www.aln.org/publications/jaln/v5n2/pdf/v5n2_brown.pdf

Buchanan, E. A., Myers, S. E., & Hardin, S. L. (2005). Holding your hand from a distance: Online mentoring and the graduate library and information sciences student [Electronic version]. *The Journal of Educators Online, 2*(2). Retrieved February 23, 2009, from the EBSCO host database.

Burgess, K. R. (2007). Mentoring as holistic online instruction [Electronic version]. *New Directions for Adult and Continuing Education, 113*, 49–56.

Douglass, L. R. (2007). Contemplative online learning environments [Electronic version]. *Journal of Online Education*. Retrieved online February 23, 2009, from http://www.nyu.edu/classes/keefer/waoe/douglass.htm

Holly, C., Legg, T., Mueller, D., & Adelman, D. S. (2008). Online teaching: Challenges for a new faculty role. *Journal of Professional Nursing, 24*(4), 224–258. Retrieved online February 25, 2009, from EBSCO host database.

Ivankova, N. V., & Stick, S. L. (2005). Collegiality and community: Building means for sustaining student persistence in the computer-mediated asynchronous learning environment. *Online Journal of Distance Learning Administration, 8*(3). Retrieved June 11, 2007, from http://www.westga.edu/~distance/ojdala/fall83/ivankova83.htm

Kreijns, K., Kirshner, P. A., Jochems, W., & Van Buuren, H. (2004). Determining sociability, social space, and social presence in asynchronous collaborative groups. *CyberPsychology & Behavior, 7*(2), 155–172. Retrieved February 15, 2009, from EBSCO host database.

Legg, T. J., Adelman, D. S., Mueller, D., & Levitt, C. (2009). Constructivist strategies in online distance education in nursing. *Journal of Nursing Education, 48*(2), 64–69.

Miller, L. C., Devaney, S. W., Kelley, G. L., & Kuehn, A. F. (2008). E-mentoring in public health nursing practice [Electronic version]. *The Journal of Continuing Education in Nursing, 39*(9), 394–399. Retrieved February 15, 2009 from EBSCO host database.

Misanchuk, M., & Anderson, T. (2001, April). *Building online community in an online environment: Communication, cooperation, and collaboration.* Paper presented at the proceedings of the Annual Mid South Technology Conference, Murfreesboro, TN. Available online at http://frank.mtsu.edu/~itconf/proceed01/19.html

Phinished.org. (2008). *About PhinisheD*. Available online at http://www.phinished.org/about.php

State University of New York–Delhi. (2008). *Online RN to BSN program*. Retrieved February 15, 2009, from http://www.delhi.edu/academics/online_degrees/nurs/index.php

Thomas, A. M. (2006). Technology: Friend or foe of mentoring relationships? In M. Orey (Ed.), *Educational and Media Yearbook* (Vol. 31, pp. 153–164). Westport, CT: Libraries Unlimited.

Tilley, D. S., Boswell, C., & Cannon, S. (2006). Developing and establishing online student learning communities. *Computers, Informatics & Nursing, 24*(3), 144–149. Retrieved September 3, 2007, from Ovid Nursing Database.

Chapter 12

A Behind-the-Scenes Look at the Faculty Role in the Online Learning Environment

Anita C. All

Administrators and faculty are striving to create cost-effective, yet attractive learning options that will improve teaching and learning. Many believe that online learning will encourage innovation and flexibility, and therefore have the potential for maximizing the use of infrastructure and resources. Differences in organizational structure and pedagogy by administrators and faculty, however, are needed as online learning is incorporated into educational programs.

The purpose of this chapter is to provide you with a behind-the-scenes look at the organizational structure and pedagogy used by faculty in the online learning environment, along with the strategies and theoretical methodologies they use to develop and design coursework. Although this chapter is slightly different than the other chapters in this book, its usefulness to you as a student should not be underestimated. Having a deeper understanding of the faculty roles and responsibilities will assist in helping you to know what to expect from your instructors and how to collaborate with them to enhance your online learning experience.

Evolving Faculty Roles

In recent years, a vision of academic institutions was to extend access to education by embracing innovative technologies such as Web-based instruction, satellite, broadcast television/cable, interactive videoconferencing, video streaming, podcasting, and audio conferencing. Despite varied opinions and hot debates, the argument that significant negative differences exist between students learning in the traditional classroom environment and students learning in the online classroom environment, where innovative technologies are a necessity, is not supported by research (Armstrong & Frueh, 2003; Russell, 1999; WCET, 2006). In fact, learning research

Embracing New Technology

In my master's program, I still hand wrote all my assignments and hired a typist. I shopped for a computer but was so overwhelmed by all the choices and my lack of knowledge that I left the store and a week later used that money to buy a horse. (I understood with the horse what I was buying and what I was getting for my dollar!) I finally did buy a computer during my PhD program, but the only advice I had on what to buy was to buy only as much as I could afford because it would be outdated the next day!

reports that distance learners perform as well or better than learners in the face-to-face environment (WCET, 2006).

The changing classroom, however, may be difficult for some faculty who remember the supercomputers that needed large rooms and controlled temperatures. That faculty did not grow up with technology or with the Internet at their fingertips. However difficult it may be, the evolving role of the faculty includes creating effective and successful learning environments by embracing new technology to meet the demands of the 21st century.

Teaching Based on Evidence

Faculty are traditionally endowed, so to speak, with numerous rights and responsibilities in an academic setting. Of these rights and responsibilities, undoubtedly the most important is the right of self-governance. Self-governance includes developing policies for behavior, student affairs, curriculum, administrative activities, and counseling students and other groups. It also involves the responsibility to evaluate curriculum, mentor students and colleagues, develop standards for promotion and tenure, and increase the numbers of doctoral prepared educators to teach and conduct research (AACN, 2006; Leners, Wilson, & Sitzman, 2007). Despite these collective responsibilities, the incorporation of up-to-date, evidence-based teaching practices remains the core responsibility of each faculty member (Finke, 2009). Consequently, individual faculty members are faced with a new paradigm shift supported by evidence-based practice that teaching be subjugated to learning. Faculty should not teach to students, but instead, they should collaborate *with* students to answer questions, solve problems, and facilitate learning (Zwirn & Muehlenkord, 2009).

Distance Delivery Methodology

As colleges and universities strive to be more marketable, they are seeking out creative and cost-effective delivery options such as distance education delivery systems. Distance education is defined in many different ways, but perhaps the broadest as "students receiving instruction in a location other than that of the faculty" (Ramsey & Clark, 2009, p. 351). Others define distance learning as a point of connection, mobile learning, and just-in-time learning (Billings, 2005).

Distance learning incorporates various methodologies and technologies and includes the use of the Internet, where students can have a world of information at their fingertips. No matter what instruction delivery method is chosen, faculty must be aware of the advantages and disadvantages of each system. Faculty, along with students, must also remember that it is not a magic solution to workload responsibilities. Faculty providing the instruction and students receiving the instruction must understand their roles and responsibilities when working within these distance delivery systems. Faculty responsibilities include organizing course material, designing activities that encourage learning of the content, and evaluating the accomplishment of course outcomes, while the student's responsibility is primarily to be an active participant in the learning process and take deliberate control for learning (Gibbons et al., 2008). The use of technology in distance education has tremendous power; however, it is necessary that colleges and universities integrate the various tools and methods into an overall plan that is based on sound educational theories and principles.

Learning Environment

Learning Environments/Spaces

Successful online environments/spaces contain participants who perceive they are connected by various methods such as online forums; blogs; social networking sites, such as Facebook; and others. If participants are to perceive a learning space rather than a social space, the online environment must support the learner in achieving understanding of the use of the setting and the context of the setting. Faculty need to provide explicit criteria to promote this behavior and interaction. In order to do this, faculty must reconceptualize the role of the teacher and the roles of the learner to be successful in educating the students of the future. The majority of generation X and generation Y students expect ready access to courses and flexibility in scheduling to meet all their educational and college experiences. This generation of students is accustomed to using technology in education and in their social lives. They participate in electronic social networking, text messaging, and twittering, and they expect the faculty to be competent in these activities.

Faculty may not have the innate skills or in many cases the acquired skills to create an effective online environment without extensive development, but the pressure to get on the train has been evident. For many faculty, online courses can have a tsunami effect, arriving quickly, stunningly, and in massive proportions, and this can lead to anxiety, uncertainty, and confusion for faculty and students (Gruendemann, 2007). Faculty must understand the delivery mechanics and acquire the necessary skills so they can give their full attention to learners rather than giving it to technology (Hylton, 2007).

> **The "Tsunami Effect"**
>
> I remember one of the first sessions I did for faculty to prepare them for teaching in the online setting. My lecture was titled, "Surviving Your First Online Course." One of the faculty members cheerfully started the session but ended up leaving in tears at the midpoint because she was so overwhelmed with the technology and software management system that she was just not ready for tips on organizing discussions, managing all the email, and so on.

Facilitating Learning

In order for interaction to occur, learners must communicate with each other. Faculty cannot assume that lack of physical presence is a barrier to social presence in an electronic

Be Careful with the Tone and Attitude of the Message

A personal issue of mine, as an online educator, is email. I like to provide very quick feedback to email and telephone messages; however, I have several email accounts. I have two university email accounts and several course email accounts, and as a result, my message centers can become overwhelming. I am often embroiled in getting messages read and answers or suggestions provided when, on some days, there can be over 100 messages. Students have given me the opportunity to improve my online communication and teaching by posting comments saying they perceive me as abrupt. Although my purpose is to get the answers out quickly, I have learned to be somewhat more social by saying, "Hi" and ending with, "Do you have more questions or ideas?" I feel all communications should be professional and written so that you do not need to worry about what your boss would think if he or she reads them. The world of text messaging and twittering is something that my learners are much more comfortable with than I am. I am working on it!

environment (Sargeant, Curran, Allen, Jarvis-Selinger, & Ho, 2006; Yen & Tu, 2008). Rogers and Lea (2005) reported that, in fact, the lack of physical presence may be an advantage to improving social presence due to emphasizing social identities versus personal identities. The social learning theory suggests that learning takes place when there is interaction with and observation of others within a social context (Sargeant et al., 2006). A high level of social presence initiates and maintains greater interaction in online courses and is positively related to the quality of knowledge acquisition, perceived learning, perceived satisfaction, and student-perceived learning achievements (Richardson & Swan, 2003; Russo & Benson, 2005). Faculty, however, cannot assume that interaction will occur, because it will not unless the faculty carefully and deliberately plan and create a social place and a social presence. One way to enhance social presence is to pay careful attention to writing style. Writing styles in the virtual world indicate expression, tone of voice, and intent. Another way to enhance social presence is to facilitate group learning. In the online learning environment, faculty can serve as facilitators of group learning by encouraging sharing and exploration and posing questions that encourage deeper understanding and critical thinking.

Implementing Online Learning

The role of facilitator, however, does not lessen the importance of the faculty role. Ultimate responsibility for course design including identification of expected outcomes, designing learning activities that will promote active student involvement, and evaluating student performance remains in the hands of the faculty (Halstead & Billings, 2009). Course design best practices (Billings, Conners, & Skiba, 2001) indicate that the design impacts how students learn and how well the course influences time on tasks and productive use of students' learning time. Best practices in the online learning environment are really basic in nature and are not different from best teaching practices in any setting. These best practices include (Distance Education Report, 2009):

- Show up and teach.
- Practice proactive course management strategies.
- Establish patterns of course activities.
- Plan for the unplanned.
- Respond when requested and/or expected.
- Think before you write.
- Help maintain forward progress.
- Be safe and secure.
- Quality counts.
- Click a mile on my connection.

Most of these practices need little if any explanation. The "respond when requested and/or expected" best practice stresses the importance of timely feedback, and this does not differ from traditional educational settings because students' academic progress can be hindered if timely feedback is not received. The "click a mile on my connection" (Distance Education Report, 2009) best practice speaks to the fact that students and faculty need access to the same technology for success. In the ideal world, some faculty have access to course design specialists (e.g., instructional designers, graphic artists, and Web technicians) (Blood-Siegfried et al., 2008; Halstead & Billings, 2009). Unfortunately, other faculty have limited resources; these faculty must often assume the responsibility for the technological design of courses, the technology involved, and the integrity of the courses.

Understand Your Role as Faculty in the Online Learning Environment

Early in our venture into online learning at one university, we were mandated to put at least 50% of each graduate course online. Some faculty development was provided, but it was primarily aimed at learning how to use the course software. One faculty member completely developed her course and loaded it on WebCT, but did not interact with the students. The students kept asking which faculty member was teaching the course. Upon further investigation I found that the faculty member never did anything except grade and return assignments. She did not understand the role she played in the online learning environment and students considered her missing in action.

Drop a Note

I found that if I get involved in many activities and I am not as active in a discussion in one module versus another, I get a lot of informal complaints from students. I have found if I drop a note to let the students know what is going on, such as, "The dean dropped a proposal in my lap and I will be somewhat absent over the next couple of days," students are really understanding and appreciate the candor.

Course Design

The role of course design needs to be emphasized. Overcoming the challenge of making technology-based courses both adaptive and inviting to student needs can prove difficult for educators when explicit and implicit degrees of separation are imposed by distance (Gibbons et al., 2008). Therefore, the success of a course starts before the students enroll. Course design is the key to building online learning communities. Six elements for incorporation into each course to promote interaction are honesty, responsiveness, relevance, respect, openness, and empowerment. Students need to know that they can expect honest, respectful, and constructive feedback and prompt response. Content needs to be relevant to program outcomes, and students need to be empowered to be self-directed. Often dividing the content into clear, distinct areas or modules leads to effective design (Gobet et al., 2001). Clear and specific guidelines for online course behaviors should be unmistakably delineated early in the course, such as, "I would expect to see you logged into the course 3 hours per week, and your participation in discussion will be graded according to guidelines for participation."

Reaching out to students in the early weeks of a course will promote success. Course design strategies such as round robin, debate, and discussion questions that require analysis, synthesis, evaluation and reflection, short written work, and collaborative group work are various methods used to engage students from diverse backgrounds to think creatively. Encouraging this type of interaction between and among students and faculty and incorporating the six elements discussed previously can assist in building a community of online learners that will seek to clarify concepts and brainstorm solutions to problems or ethical issues.

> **Reaching Out to Students**
>
> In a large nursing theory class I had a student who was, according to the course tracking tool, constantly logging into the course, but was not participating. I sent an email to the student in the second week on both the course email system and the university system, and when I did not receive a response from the student I sent a second email. I did not hear from the student so I called her. She was thankful for the call because she knew she was missing course material but she thought since the course was online that she could not call!

Course Effectiveness

Several methods may be used by faculty to enhance course effectiveness. These may include (Halstead & Billings, 2009):

- Consistent design format to organize courses
- Course design that promotes ease of navigation and interaction
- Consistent methods of communication
- A few carefully designed assignments that encourage practice
- Prompt feedback

- Feedback from other students
- Sampling of graded assignments (not usually favored by students)
- Grading rubrics
- Small discussion groups

Small Groups

A colleague and I had many interesting conversations on how to use small groups. He maintained the same groups throughout the course, and I changed membership with each discussion question/module. His thoughts were that learning was facilitated by maintaining the same groups for discussions while my thought was that changing the groups was better at facilitating learning. We were both right but it is imperative to look at the purpose of the small groups, type of course, and course objectives when deciding what strategy to use.

Evaluating Outcomes

No matter the distance modality, evaluation is important in terms of students and program outcomes. Reports of best practices (Blood-Siegfried et al., 2008; Gibbons et al., 2008; Halstead & Billings, 2009; Jackson & Helms, 2008) point out that evaluation begins with clearly stated and communicated learning outcomes/competencies, providing students with an opportunity to practice the expected behaviors and receive feedback during the learning process. The reports also state that grading should indicate the degree to which learning has occurred. These aspects of evaluation are not different from what faculty does when teaching in a face-to-face traditional classroom setting. The outcomes and how learners get there should be specific and transparent to the learners.

Course faculty need to be deliberate and conscious in the timing of evaluations. A great deal of thought needs to be given in choosing evaluation strategies and providing feedback during the course. For example, if you know you have an out-of-town conference and you know you will not provide feedback for 2 weeks, do not make a paper due just before you leave. Be sure that formative evaluation, or feedback at points along the way, is part of your strategy. Provide opportunities for students to practice in order to assure understanding.

Concept or Cognitive Maps

I have found that the teaching/learning strategy of creating concept or cognitive maps is useful from both a learner and facilitator view. These maps, or visual representations, provide a very visual depiction for understanding and can be used by students to ferret out the key ideas in readings and discussions. I use concept mapping as a developmental series when asking students to do concept analysis.

Occasionally, discussion on the muddiest point will help during the course. It can be used to move forward on specific course issues as well as in subsequent course revisions. Summative evaluation, or evaluation at the end of the course that looks at overall accomplishment of outcomes, is useful depending on course content. A review of all course material, if a comprehensive evaluation is utilized, can include written work, games, debates, discussion, portfolios, electronic poster presentations, and tests. Students will usually express gratitude for reviews before a summative evaluation. As a side note, faculty should take advantage of course management tools, such as online grade books, in order to work effectively and efficiently. These online tools provide timely feedback that assists students in keeping track of their own progress.

Course Integrity

Integrity in the academic setting continues to be a priority no matter what the delivery method. If there are no academic honesty or dishonesty policies in writing, they need to be developed. The electronic environment and the Internet provide new opportunities for access to papers and projects worldwide from students. In addition, many violations of plagiarism can occur when students do not understand all the conventions of citations. Methods such as honor codes, selectively alternating assignments, and offering information on how to properly cite references can also be useful. Expensive and complicated detection software is also available to check written work for similarities. Some specific suggestions (WCET, 2008) to promote academic integrity are:

- Use of multiple assessment techniques in place of high-stakes exams
- Greater reliance on written assignments and threaded discussion
- Use of test banks and timed test delivery
- Raising awareness among students about what constitutes appropriate and inappropriate academic behavior in an online course
- Plagiarism detection software and browser lockdowns
- Physical proctoring centers for exam delivery
- Remote proctoring devices
- Other student identity technologies

It is important to note that students can still cheat and really are very inventive when determined to cheat. Face-to-face courses now have trouble with microrecorders in test reviews and smart phones that take pictures of the examination. A student determined to cheat may succeed in doing so. On the whole, those experienced in online teaching do not relate greater differences in cheating for online courses versus traditional classroom courses (WCET, 2008).

Faculty can use academic honesty policies positively by facilitating discussions of what plagiarism is and what it means to you if you were the author, why integrity matters in the future, and what potential employers expect. Examples and case studies that highlight issues and ethical concerns of honesty can serve to be valuable learning experiences and rich online discussions for students.

Conclusion

It cannot be overstated that the online classroom is an increasingly popular alternative to the traditional classroom setting. Developing online courses and engaging diverse students and faculty in the e-learning process requires creativity, adaptability, and flexibility. Students who have a deeper understanding of what happens behind the scenes in an online course will be better prepared to function and succeed in this environment.

Sample Checklist for Faculty Planning

_______ Decide course purpose

_______ Decide course objectives

_______ Consult instructional design specialists

_______ Reconceptualize course material

_______ Decide course layout

_______ Investigate common course navigation tools

_______ Decide degree of student interaction and evaluation

_______ Develop grading criteria or rubrics

_______ Sign up for technology training

_______ Load course into course management system

References

American Association of Colleges of Nursing (AACN). (2006). *Nurse educator report.* New York: Author.

Armstrong, M., & Frueh, S. (2003). *Telecommunications for nurses: Providing successful distance education and telehealth* (2nd ed.). New York: Springer.

Billings, D. M. (2005). From teaching to learning in a mobile wired world [Guest editorial]. *Journal of Nursing Education, 44,* 343.

Billings, D., Conners, H., & Skiba, D. (2001). Benchmarking best practices in Web-based nursing courses. *Advances in Nursing Science, 23*(3), 41–52.

Blood-Siegfried, J. E., Short, N. M., Rapp, C. G., Hill, E., Talbert, S., Skinner, J., et al. (2008). A rubric for improving the quality of online courses. *International Journal of Nursing Education Scholarship, 5*(1), 1–13.

DeBourge, G. A. (2003). Predictors of student satisfaction in distance-delivered graduate nursing courses: What matters most? *Journal of Professional Nursing, 19,* 149–163.

Distance Education Report. (2009). *10 principles of effective online teaching: Best practices in distance education.* Retrieved June 17, 2009, from http://www.facultyfocus.com/free-report/10-effective-classroom-management-techniques-every-faculty-member-should-know

Finke, L. M. (2009). Teaching in nursing: The faculty role. In D. M. Billings & J. A. Halstead, *Teaching in nursing: A guide for faculty* (3rd ed., pp. 3–17). St. Louis, MO: Saunders Elsevier.

Gibbons, A. S., Merrill, P. F., Swan, R., Campbell, J. O., Christensen, E., Insalaco, M., et al. (2008). Reexamining the implied role of the designer. *The Quarterly Review of Distance Education, 9*(2), 127–137.

Gobet, F., Lane, P. C. R., Croker, S., Cheng, P. C. H., Jones, G., Oliver, I., et al. (2001). Chunking mechanisms in human learning. *Trends in Cognitive Science, 5*(6), 236–243.

Gruendemann, B. J. (2007). Distance learning and perioperative nursing. *AORN Journal, 85*(3), 574–586.

Halstead, J. A., & Billings, D. M. (2009). Teaching and learning in online learning communities. In D. M. Billings & J. A. Halstead (Eds.), *Teaching in nursing: A guide for faculty* (3rd ed., pp. 369–387). St. Louis, MO: Saunders Elsevier.

Hylton, M. E. (2007). Facilitating online learning communities: A comparison of two discussion facilitation techniques. *Journal of Technology in Human Services, 25*(4), 63–78.

Jackson, M. J., & Helms, M. M. (2008, September/October). Students' perceptions of hybrid courses: Measuring and interpreting quality. *Journal of Education for Business,* 7–12.

Leners, D. W., Wilson, V. W., & Sitzman, K. L. (2007). Twenty-first century doctoral education: Online with a focus on nursing education. *Nursing Education Perspectives, 28*(6), 332–336.

Ramsey, R. W., & Clark, C. E. (2009). Teaching and learning at a distance. In D. M. Billings & J. A. Halstead (Eds.), *Teaching in nursing: A guide for faculty* (3rd ed.). St. Louis, MO: Saunders Elsevier.

Richardson, J. C., & Swan, K. (2003). Examining social presence in online courses in relation to students' perceived learning and satisfaction. *Journal of Asynchronous Learning Networks, 7*(1), 68–88.

Rogers, P., & Lea, M. (2005). Social presence in distributed group environments: The role of social identity. *Behaviour & Information Technology, 24*(2), 151–158.

Russell, T. L. (1999). *The no significant difference phenomenon: A comparative research annotated bibliography for technology for distance education*. Montgomery, AL: International Distance Education Certification Center.

Russo, T., & Benson, S. (2005). Learning with invisible others: Perceptions of online presence and their relationship to cognitive and affective learning. *Educational Technology & Society, 8*(1), 54–62.

Sargeant, J., Curran, V., Allen, M., Jarvis-Selinger, S., & Ho, K. (2006). Facilitating interpersonal interaction and learning online: Linking theory to practice. *Journal of Continuing Education in Health Professions, 26*(2), 128–136.

Swan, K., & Shih, L. F. (2005). On the nature and development of social presence in online course discussions. *Journal of Asynchronous Learning Networks, 9*(3), Retrieved April 25, 2009, from http://www.sloan-c.org/publications/jaln/index.asp?op0=OR&filter0%5B%5D=145

WCET. (2006). *No significant difference phenomenon*. Retrieved June 13, 2009, from http://nosignificantdifference.wcet.info

WCET. (2008). *Are your online students really the ones registered for the course?* Retrieved June 13, 2009, from http://wiche.edu/attachment_library/Briefing_Paper_Feb_2008.pdf

Yen, C-J., & Tu, C-H. (2008). Online social presence: A study of score validity of the computer-mediated communication questionnaire. *Quarterly Review of Distance Education, 9*(3), 297–310.

Zwirn, E. E., & Muehlenkord, A. (2009). Using media, multimedia, and technology rich environments. In D. M. Billings & J. A. Halstead (Eds.), *Teaching in nursing: A guide for faculty* (3rd ed., pp. 335–350). St. Louis, MO: Saunders Elsevier.

Technology Defined

Chad Troxell and Michael R. George

A

Adobe Reader Adobe Reader is a free program created and distributed by Adobe Systems. Once downloaded, the program can be used to view, print, and search PDF files but it cannot create or edit PDF files (Adobe Systems, Inc., 2009b).

Asynchronous learning Asynchronous learning is a student-centered teaching method that does not require all parties to be present at the same time. Instead, information is posted at a specific posting site for the parties to read and respond to at their convenience.

Atomic Learning Atomic Learning is a subscription-based service that offers thousands of short tutorial movies and educational resources to answer software and technology questions (Atomic Learning, 2009).

Attachment An attachment is a document or file that accompanies an email.

Audacity Audacity is free, open-source software for recording and editing audio files (Audacity, n.d.).

B

Bandwidth Bandwidth is the amount of data that can be transmitted in a fixed amount of time. For digital devices the bandwidth is usually expressed in bits per second or bytes per second. For analog devices, the bandwidth is expressed in cycles per second, or hertz (Hz).

Blackboard Blackboard is an online learning course management system that allows faculty to transmit information to students including, but not limited to, the class syllabus, faculty contact information, class schedules, assignments, and announcements.

Bookmark A bookmark is feature built into Internet browsers that allows the user to collect and organize Web sites so they can be easily found at a later point in time.

Bytes/second Bytes/second is the amount of bit rate or data transfer rate. This is most commonly measured in kilobytes per second (KB/s) or megabytes per second (MB/s).

C

Camtasia Camtasia is a video-based screen capturing software program. It is analogous to using a video camera to record your computer screen and it can be used with or without voice narration. Camtasia has been used to deliver live presentations, lectures, software tutorials, narrated PowerPoint presentations, narrated lecture notes and homework, video and audio podcast production, and more (TechSmith Corporation, 2009a).

Crazy Talk Crazy Talk is a software program that can transform photos and images into talking animated characters and bring them to life with real-time puppeteering (Reallusion, 2009).

Creative commons license A creative commons license protects the work developed by individuals. It grants permission to other people to copy and distribute the work providing they give credit to the individual who developed the work. A creative commons license is identified by double Cs (CC) (Creative Commons, n.d.).

D

Discussion forum The discussion forum within the online learning classroom provides students and faculty with a virtual forum for professional collaboration, dialogue, brainstorming along with practicing new skills, strategies, and applying new knowledge.

Discussion threads Discussion threads, also called topic threads or threaded discussions, group together messages in the discussion forum that share a common subject heading.

Distance e-learning Distance e-learning is a Web-based teaching strategy used to deliver information and facilitate learning in a virtual classroom. All communications are mediated by some type of electronic means in either real time (synchronous) or delayed time (asynchronous).

E

Eduspace Eduspace is an online learning course management system that provides course management tools and text-specific content to make it easy for instructors to teach all or part of a course online (Cengage Learning, n.d.).

Electronic portfolio An electronic portfolio is an electronic collection and storage of documents, images, photos, audio, and more. It is analogous to a traditional portfolio except that the information is stored electronically.

Email (electronic mail) Email is a method of sending mail electronically through an Internet- or network-based service.

F

Facebook Facebook is an online social networking forum. It enables users to share information and keep up with friends, colleagues, and classmates. Registration is required but it is free (Facebook, 2009).

FAST FAST is a free online assessment survey tool that can be used to obtain a summary of the students' impressions of a course and/or the students' impressions of a teacher. It not only tracks numbers, but it enables the user to collect valuable qualitative comments while maintaining anonymity (FAST, 2004).

Feed aggregator A feed aggregator, also known as a feed reader, is an application that allows users to subscribe to multiple syndicated news feeds and read them in one place.

Flash Flash, developed by Adobe Systems, is a file format used to deliver video and interactive content over the Internet. Flash files have a file extension of SWF or FLV.

Flickr Flickr is an online photo management and sharing application that enables the user to upload, edit, organize, and share photos and videos (Flickr, 2009). Some images in Flickr are under a creative commons license (see "creative commons"), while others are considered to be public domain (see "public domain").

G

Garage Band Garage Band is a software application that allows users to create music or insert music into podcasts (Apple, Inc., 2009).

Google Apps Google Apps are Web applications used to assist in enhancing Web-based communication, collaboration, and security for work, school, or business. Examples of Google Apps include Google Talk (users can call and instant message friends through a computer), Google Docs (allows users to share online documents, presentations, and spreadsheets), and Google Calendar (users organize schedules and share events with friends) (Google Apps, 2009).

H

HTML (hypertext markup language) HTML is a type of text code that, when embedded in a document, allows the document to be read and distributed across the Internet.

Hybrid course A hybrid course is a blend of face-to-face instruction and distance learning.

Hyperlink A hyperlink is a text, image, and/or graphic that will connect the user to a Web page or to another place in the same document when activated by a click of the mouse or a keystroke. The hyperlink is usually underlined and is frequently in blue.

I

Impatica for PowerPoint Impatica for PowerPoint is software that delivers fully narrated and highly animated PowerPoint presentations to any Internet device without the use of plug-ins. It does this by converting the PowerPoint file into a compressed format for streaming over the Internet. Impatica is compatible with Blackboard, WebCT, and eCollege (Impatica, 2009).

Internet The Internet, in simplest terms, allows people from around the world to connect and share a plethora of information through the computer.

J

Java Runtime Java Runtime is a programming language that has its own unique programming tools and technologies. Java works with an Internet browser to allow users to play online games, view 3D images, and create interactive online experiences (Sun Microsystems, Inc., 2009).

JPEG (Joint Photographic Experts Group) JPEG is a compressed image file format used for compressing photographic images. The files' extensions are JPEG and JPG.

L

Learning communities Learning communities are communities that are formed when a group of students, instructors, and/or mentors sharing similar subjects, classes, coursework, or majors come together to collaborate and learn from one another. See "online collegiality."

Learning management system Learning management systems (LMSs) are electronic classrooms that can be accessed by individuals who are registered and have a password. Examples of LMSs include Blackboard, WebCT, and Eduspace (Kameron, 2003).

LinkedIn LinkedIn is a professional networking site where people from around the world can exchange knowledge, ideas, and opportunities (LinkedIn Corporation, 2009).

LISTSERV LISTSERV is an electronic mailing list made of up email addresses, and the lists are defined by groups of common interests.

M

MERLOT (Multimedia Educational Resource for Learning and Online Teaching) MERLOT is an online educational resource site that contains a collection of peer-reviewed teaching and learning materials. Membership is required, but it is free (MERLOT, 2009).

Microsoft Office Microsoft Office is a software suite of different applications that include Microsoft Word, Microsoft PowerPoint, Microsoft Excel, Microsoft Access, and Microsoft Publisher (Microsoft Corporation, 2009).

MP3 (MPEG-1 Audio Layer-3) MP3 is a compressed audio file format that digitizes music for downloading onto a digital music player such as an iPod.

MySpace MySpace is a free social networking Web site where members can create a profile, share in-depth information about personal interests, and designate how they want this information to be shared with others. Registration is free (MySpace.com, 2009).

N

Netiquette Netiquette is the rules of etiquette that are to be followed when communicating by computer.

O

Online collegiality Online collegiality is the development of social relationships in an online environment as a result of sharing a course of study together for a given period of time. See "learning communities."

Open source Open source refers to any program whose source code is available for use or modification. Generally the programs are available free of charge.

P

PDF PDF (portable document format) is a distribution format created by Adobe Systems that enables information to be transferred electronically between computers (Adobe Systems, Inc., 2009a).

Plain text Plain text is based on the English language alphabet and consists of 26 lower case and 26 upper case letters as well as Arabic numerals and various punctuation marks. The plain text format does not support any type of text formatting, such as italics, underlining, or varying font sizes or colors; however, it is an efficient method of storing text because it takes up less than half the size of rich text documents consisting of identical characters (The Linux Information Project, 2007; Swift, n.d.). See "RTF (rich text format)."

Podcast A podcast is an online audio broadcast that has been converted to an MP3 file or other audio file format for playback in a digital music player. Although podcasts are mostly verbal, they may contain music, images, and video (NotePage, Inc., 2009; PCMAG, n.d.).

Podcatcher A podcatcher captures an RSS feed (see "RSS") and posts it to a site where it automatically downloads a podcast onto a subscriber's computer or mobile device. Once downloaded, subscribers to the RSS feed can then listen to the podcast at their convenience (Indiana University, 2007).

Public domain Any item that is classified as public domain is public property and does not require a citation, permission of use, or royalties. Public domain is anything that is not covered by copyright or creative commons licenses.

R

Response system A response system, personal response system (PRS), or student's response system (SRS) allows large groups of people to vote on a topic or answer questions. Each person has a remote control with which selections can be made. Quizdom and TurningPoint are two examples of response systems.

RSS RSS is an abbreviation for *really simple syndication* or *rich site summary*. A content provider publishes a feed link, RSS feed, on its site, to which users can subscribe. The feed content then can be redisplayed and automatically updated by any user by using a feed aggregator or widget.

RTF (rich text format) Rich text is a higher grade of text than plain text in that it does support italics, underlining, varying font sizes, font colors, and various styles of page formatting. Documents in rich text, therefore, require more computer space when saving compared to the documents in plain text (see "plain text").

S

SCORM SCORM (shareable content object reference model) is a framework used to set technical programming standards for e-learning software products to ensure the products can be easily shared among different learning management systems. SCORM was developed in response to the United States Department of Defense initiative to promote standardization in e-learning (SearchSOA.com, 2002).

Screen cast A screen cast is a digital recording of part or all of the computer screen output. Screen casts can include an audio narration and are useful for demonstrating how to accomplish a task on the computer.

Second Life Second Life is a free 3D virtual world imagined and created by its residents. Individuals are able to walk, teleport, or even fly to thousands of exciting 3D locations. One can also use voice and text chat to communicate with other real people from around the world (Second Life, 2009).

Snagit Snagit is a screen capture software program that allows users to take high-quality snapshots of anything on their computer screen (TechSmith Corporation, 2009b).

Social networking Social networking is a group of people coming together online to share common interests. These people often have similar backgrounds, hobbies, political ideas, or any factors that would bring people together in a forum to socialize and interact. Facebook and MySpace are two examples of social networking groups (What is Social Networking.com, 2009).

Streaming audio/video Streaming audio (sound)/video (pictures) are computer files that immediately play in their entirety once opened by the computer user. The media is transmitted continuously without the user having to download it (Tech Target, 2008).

Synchronous learning Synchronous learning is a student-centered teaching method that occurs when all parties are present at the same time to discuss and share information.

T

Turnitin Turnitin is an Internet-based plagiarism-detection service created by iParadigms, LLC (iParadigms LLC, 2009).

Twitter Twitter is a friend-of-a-friend social networking site designed for friends, families, and coworkers to stay connected. Twitter is defined by the short, 140-character messages, also know as "tweets," that can be posted and reposted on followers' pages (Twitter, 2009).

U

URL (uniform resource locators) A URL is a method of locating and accessing online resources. A URL commonly begins with http, https, or ftp and is followed by information that will direct the user to a file or a specific program.

V

Virtual classroom A virtual classroom is a simulated or conceptual classroom. It is not physical in nature. In distance learning, the virtual classroom serves as the forum for online communication and collaboration between students and instructors.

Virtual chalkboard A virtual chalkboard is an electronic teaching tool used to video capture text that is written on a computer screen, otherwise know as screen casting.

Virtual chalkboard lecture A virtual chalkboard lecture is a video capture of what the instructor is writing on the chalkboard. If audio is used, students can hear the instructors lecture as they watch the video.

W

Web 2.0 The term "Web 2.0" refers to a perceived second generation of Web development and design that aims to facilitate communication, secure information sharing, and enhance collaboration on the World Wide Web (O'Reilly, 2005).

Web conferencing Web conferencing is conferencing that occurs over the Internet. It can serve as a replacement for face-to-face meetings, and, because it occurs over the Internet, it is one solution that can assist in enhancing the ability to exchange ideas and information with colleagues and business partners from all over the world (Osborn, 2005). Examples of Web conferencing sites are Yugma, GoToMeeting, and DimDim.

Widget A widget is code that can be embedded within a Web page, and it produces nonstatic content. Widgets can provide information in the form of RSS feed readers, clocks, or weather forecasts.

Y

YouTube YouTube is a social site that allows people to easily upload and share video clips across the Internet through Web sites, mobile devices, blogs, and email (YouTube, LLC, 2009).

Z

ZIP files ZIP files are compressed files that are used to reduce the overall size of the included file(s), reduce the amount of disk space needed for storage, and reduce download times. In order to view the contents of a ZIP file, the user needs to upzip or uncompress the file (Microsoft Corporation, 2007).

References

Adobe Systems, Inc. (2009a). *Adobe and PDF.* Retrieved July 16, 2009, from http://www.adobe.com/products/acrobat/adobepdf.html

Adobe Systems, Inc. (2009b). *Product comparison.* Retrieved July 15, 2009, from http://www.adobe.com/products/acrobat/matrix.html

Apple, Inc. (2009). *iLife 09.* Retrieved June 11, 2009, from Apple Store (U.S.), http://store.apple.com/us/product/MB966Z/A/iLife-09

Atomic Learning, Inc. (2009). *Atomic learning.* Retrieved May 1, 2009, from http://movies.atomiclearning.com/k12/home

Audacity. (n.d.). *The free, cross-platform sound editor.* Retrieved June 25, 2009, from http://audacity.sourceforge.net

Cengage Learning. (n.d.). *Eduspace—online learning tool.* Retrieved May 4, 2009, from http://www.cengage.com/eduspace

Creative Commons. (n.d.). *License your work.* Retrieved July 14, 2009, from http://creativecommons.org/license

Facebook. (2009). *About Facebook.* Retrieved April 10, 2009, from http://www.facebook.com/facebook?ref=pf

FAST. (2004). *Free assessment summary tool.* Retrieved April 1, 2009, from http://www.getfast.ca

Flickr. (2009). *What is Flickr?* Retrieved May 4, 2009, from http://www.flickr.com/tour

Google Apps. (2009). *Join over a million businesses saving time and money.* Retrieved July 14, 2009, from http://www.google.com/apps/intl/en/business/index.html

Impatica. (2009). *Impatica for PowerPoint.* Retrieved June 25, 2009, from http://www.impatica.com/imp4ppt

Indiana University. (2007). *What is a podcatcher?* Retrieved April 1, 2009 from http://kb.iu.edu/data/auej.html

iParadigms LLC. (2009). *Metrics on the effectiveness of Turnitin.* Retrieved July 16, 2009, from http://turnitin.com/static/effectiveness.html

Kameron, S. (2003). *Online classrooms for free?! A review of free online learning management systems (LMS).* Retrieved April 4, 2009, from http://www-writing.berkeley.edu/tesl-ej/ej26/m2.html

LinkedIn Corporation. (2009). *What is LinkedIn?* Retrieved April 1, 2009, from http://learn.linkedin.com/what-is-linkedin

The Linux Information Project. (2007). *Plain text definition.* Retreived July 14, 2009, from http://www.linfo.org/plain_text.html

MERLOT. (2009). *Welcome to MERLOT.* Retrieved April 1, 2009, from http://www.merlot.org/merlot/index.htm

Microsoft Corporation. (2007). *Description of zip (.zip) files.* Retrieved June 11, 2009, from Microsoft Help and Support, http://support.microsoft.com/kb/259177

Microsoft Corporation. (2009). *2007 Microsoft Office system suites overview.* Retrieved June 8, 2009, from Microsoft Office Suites, http://office.microsoft.com/en-us/suites/HA101757031033.aspx

MySpace.com. (2009). *Get started on MySpace.* Retrieved July 15, 2009, from http://www.myspace.com

NotePage, Inc. (2009). *What is podcasting?* Retrieved July 15, 2009, from http://www.podcasting-tools.com/what-is-podcasting.htm

O'Reilly, T. (2005). *What is Web 2.0. Design patterns and business models for the next generation of software.* Retrieved July 15, 2009, from http://oreilly.com/web2/archive/what-is-web-20.html

Osborn, A. (2005). *What is web conferencing and why has it become integral in today's business world.* Retrieved April 4, 2009, from Web-Conferencing-Zone.com Web site: http://www.web-conferencing-zone.com/what-is-web-conferencing.htm

PCMAG. (n.d.). *Encyclopedia*. Retrieved July 14, 2009, from http://www.pcmag.com/encyclopedia_term/0,2542,t=podcast&i=49433,00.asp

Reallusion. (2009). *CrazyTalk6*. Retrieved May 4, 2009, from http://www.reallusion.com/crazytalk

SearchSOA.com. (2002). *Shareable content object reference model*. Retrieved July 14, 2009, from http://searchsoa.techtarget.com/sDefinition/0,,sid26_gci796793,00.html

Second Life. (2009). *What is Second Life?* Retrieved July 13, 2009, from http://secondlife.com/whatis

Sun Microsystems, Inc. (2009). *New to Java programming center*. Retrieved July 15, 2009, from http://java.sun.com/new2java

Swift, J. (n.d.). *ASCII: What is it and why should I care?* Retrieved July 15, 2009, from http://www.telacommunications.com/nutshell/ascii.htm

TechSmith Corporation. (2009a). *Camtasia Studio*. Retrieved July 13, 2009 from http://www.techsmith.com/camtasia.asp

TechSmith Corporation. (2009b). *Snagit product tour*. Retrieved June 12, 2009, from http://www.techsmith.com/learn/snagit/getting-started/default.asp

Tech Target. (2008). *Streaming media*. Retrieved July 14, 2009, from http://whatis.techtarget.com/definition/0,,sid9_gci753540,00.html

Twitter. (2009). *What is Twitter*? Retrieved July 15, 2009, from http://www.twitter.com

What is Social Networking.com. (2009). *What is social networking?* Retrieved July 14, 2009, from http://www.whatissocialnetworking.com

YouTube, LLC. (2009). *Company history*. Retrieved June 8, 2009, from http://www.youtube.com/t/about

Appendix A

Online Learning: Myths Versus Reality

Stacia Thompson

Myth	Reality
Online learning can be done at your own pace.	Although online learning can take place any time and any place with Internet connectivity, most courses have strict deadlines that must be met.
Online learning is easy.	Online learning is student centered and places much of the responsibility for learning on the student.
Online learning takes place on your own with little interaction.	Online learning requires a great deal of interaction between student and teacher as well as among students.
All online courses are the same.	Online learning opportunities vary from self-paced learning modules to fully interactive virtual classrooms.
Online learning takes less time.	Online learning may actually require a greater time commitment but results in an increased learning potential.

Appendix B

Study Strategies

Stacia Thompson

- *S*urvey, *Q*uestion, *R*ead, *R*ecite, and *R*eview (Cook Counseling Center at Virginia Tech [CCC], 2000). This is called the SQ3R technique, and it can be used each time you read new material.
- Do not hesitate to write in your books. Highlight what is important and what needs further exploration.
- Keep a dictionary, thesaurus, and APA manual handy. Look up words you do not know and write out the definitions.

Reference

Cook Counseling Center at Virginia Tech (CCC). (2000). *Increasing textbook comprehension by using SQ3R.* Retrieved December 31, 2008 from http://www.ucc.vt.edu/lynch/TextbookReading.htm

Appendix C

Students in the Military: Is an Online Learning Program a Viable Option?

Stacia Thompson

Plan ahead	· What are your postmilitary plans? · Are you planning on working on a degree? · Where do you want to go to school?
Take the initiative	· Check out the availability of online courses. · Look at the college you plan to attend upon discharge. · What does that college offer online that you could start on now? · Check out the resources offered at your assigned duty station. There may be counselors to help you plan an educational program to meet your needs.
Advantages	· With the frequent moves made by persons in the military, you may not have to change institutions, and you may be able to complete your entire degree online no matter where you are stationed.
Connectivity	· Investigate with your superiors the availability of computer connectivity.
Communication	· Communicate with your instructor about your situation. · If you are deployed to a remote location, you may have to make arrangements to complete some assignments in an alternative format.

Appendix D

Taking Multiple Courses at One Time: Do I Have Enough Time in the Day?

Stacia Thompson

Evaluate the need for multiple courses	· Why are you planning to take more than one course at a time? · Is it absolutely necessary?
Consider other demands on your time	· What other responsibilities do you have? · Are there enough hours in the day to devote adequate time to multiple courses while meeting other responsibilities?
Support available	· What support do you have to help with other responsibilities? · Are you willing to delegate some of your responsibilities to others? · Are others willing to accept these responsibilities?
Time management skills	· How good are you at managing your time? · How good are your study habits, writing skills, and computer skills? · Set up a time schedule, before committing to multiple courses, to assess if there is enough time in the day to complete the additional coursework.

Appendix E

Check Into Employee Tuition Reimbursement

Julie Fomenko

Do not neglect to look into tuition reimbursement options provided by your employer. "More than 50% of employers with 100-plus employees offer some type of tuition reimbursement in their benefit packages" (eLearners.com, 2008, para. 4). If tuition reimbursement is offered by your employer, many, if not all of the costs associated with your class or your entire program could be covered.

Reference

eLearners.com. (2008). *You are ready to go back to school if . . .* Retrieved January 24, 2009, from http://www.elearners.com/guide-to-online-education/you-are-ready-to-go-back-to-school.asp?nl=6

Appendix F

Convenience Is a Benefit of Online Learning

Desiree Carter

The flexibility of scheduling and the ability to work and study at one's own pace anywhere in the world are major reasons that online education is so appealing (Christianson, Tiene, & Luft, 2002; Holly, Legg, Mueller, & Adelman, 2008; Pullen, 2006; Ryan, Carlton, & Ali, 2004; Singh & Pan, 2004; Travale, 2007). Students with families, jobs, and other obligations can complete their work in the early morning hours or on a lunch break. Students who lead transient lives, such as military personnel and their family members, are able to take the program with them if they move (Lorenzetti, 2005). If a student has a laptop, he or she can take the class and go outside to enjoy pleasant weather, and, with the invention of air cards, computers are capable of accessing the Internet wherever there is cell phone reception so students are even able to go on vacation and not miss a single class!

While there are still absolute due dates and deadlines that must be met, the online learning environment enables students to take whatever time is necessary in order to grasp a concept. If the learning activity includes watching a video, for example, it can be repeated until the student is thoroughly comfortable with the concept. If the student is a fast learner, he or she may be able to complete the assignments much more quickly and then finish early. The conveniences of taking online classes anywhere, anytime, and at one's own pace open the doors for educational advancement to people from all over the world.

References

Christianson, L., Tiene, D., & Luft, P. (2002). Web-based teaching in undergraduate nursing programs [Electronic version]. *Nurse Educator*, 27(6), 276–282.

Holly, C., Legg, T. J., Mueller, D., & Adelman, D. S. (2008). Online teaching: Challenges for a new faculty role. *Journal of Professional Nursing*, 24(4), 254–258.

Lorenzetti, J. P. (2005). Beyond multiple choice: Assessment for online learning. *Distance Education Report*, 9(18), 1, 6–7. Retrieved February 11, 2007, from EBSCOHost-ASP.

Pullen, D. L. (2006). An evaluative case study of online learning for healthcare professionals [Electronic version]. *The Journal of Continuing Education in Nursing*, 37(5), 225–232.

Ryan, M., Carlton, K. H., & Ali, N. S. (2004). Reflections on the role of faculty in distance learning and changing pedagogies [Electronic version]. *Nursing Education Perspectives*, 25(2), 73–80.

Singh, P., & Pan, W. (2004). Online education: Lessons for administrators and instructors [Electronic version]. *College Student Journal*, 38(2), 302–308.

Travale, I. L. (2007). Computer-assisted instruction for novice nurses in critical care [Electronic version]. *The Journal of Continuing Education in Nursing*, 38(3), 132–138.

Appendix G

Interactive Learning Is a Benefit of Online Education

Desiree Carter

Online learning is highly interactive. Christianson, Tiene, and Luft (2002) found that interaction among students actually increased in the online learning environment. This interaction can assist in enhancing communication skills, enhancing the learners' knowledge, and allowing the learner to consider ideas and opinions from varied perspectives. It can also assist in building a scholarly community among students. Although there is no face-to-face interaction in the online learning environment, students who participate in discussions and chats can quickly develop a rapport with other students that can lead to both professional and personal relationships outside of the classroom.

Developing Personal Relationships

In my program, I found that I developed many relationships with other students with whom I interacted. We often found ourselves to have many things in common and we began emailing each other outside of class on an informal basis. Some of these friendships have flourished and we still keep in touch and visit one another other on occasion to this day.

Reference

Christianson, L., Tiene, D., & Luft, P. (2002). Web-based teaching in undergraduate nursing programs [Electronic version]. *Nurse Educator*, 27(6), 276–282.

Appendix H

Field Experiences

Desiree Carter

Some online programs require students to gain practical experience in their field of study. This generally requires the student to find both a location and a mentor to supervise the learning experience and to evaluate the student performance. These experiences are often called a practicum or a field experience, and the mentor is sometimes referred to as a site supervisor.

Field Experience

I fulfilled the requirements for my field experience at a community college campus where I had been previously employed as faculty. It was much less stressful for me to be able to complete the experience there than it would have been had I been required to develop a rapport with faculty members and administrators from a different college.

Once selected, the site supervisor is usually asked to complete paperwork that verifies his or her credentials and acknowledges that he or she understands and accepts the responsibilities and expectations associated with the site supervisor role. Finding a site supervisor, however, may be problematic if the student does not have a relationship with anyone in the community who will be willing or able to serve in this capacity. If the student enrolls in a program with this type of assignment, it is crucial that the student learn the specific requirements as early in the program as possible in order to allow time for advanced planning. It is also important to determine if it is acceptable to use the location and the staff where the student is employed, as some programs will not allow students to complete their field experiences at their workplace. This would necessitate the student finding an alternative location for the learning experience.

Index